BREAKTHROUGH

JACK ANDRAKA is the recipient of the Smithsonian American Ingenuity Award, first place in the Siemens We Can Change the World Challenge, a National Geographic Explorer grant, the Intel Gordon Moore Award, and the Stockholm Water Prize. In 2013, he was Michelle Obama's personal guest at the State of the Union address. Andraka has been featured in several documentaries, including Morgan Spurlock's *You Don't Know Jack*, and in newspapers and magazines around the world. He lives in Baltimore, Maryland, and enjoys kayaking and watching *Glee*.

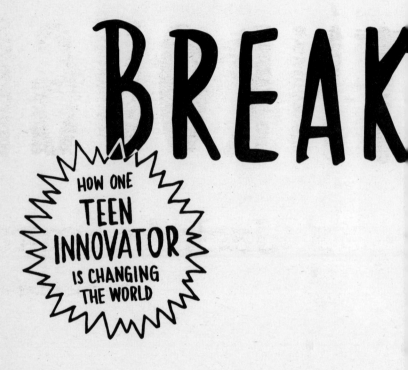

BREAK

HOW ONE
TEEN
INNOVATOR
IS CHANGING
THE WORLD

THROUGH

Jack Andraka

with
Matthew Lysiak

SCRIBE
Melbourne • London

AUTHOR'S NOTE

*Some names and identifying details have
been changed to protect the privacy of individuals.*

Scribe Publications
18–20 Edward St, Brunswick, Victoria 3056, Australia
2 John St, Clerkenwell, London, WC1N 2ES, United Kingdom

Published in the UK by Scribe 2015
First published in the United States by HarperCollins Publishers, 2015

Printed and bound in the UK by CPI Group (UK) Ltd, Croydon CR0 4YY

National Library of Australia Cataloguing-in-Publication data: Andraka, Jack, author.
Breakthrough: how one teen innovator is changing the world / Jack Andraka. 1. Andraka, Jack. 2. Scientists–Biography. 3. Cancer–Research. 4. Medical innovations. 610.92
ISBN 9781922247926 (UK edition)

Typography by Ellice M. Lee
❖

scribepublications.co.uk
scribepublications.com.au

To my **mother**, Jane;
my **father**, Steve;
and my **brother**, Luke,
whose love and support
helped me through this journey

CONTENTS

BREAKTHROUGH

From: ▐█████████████

To: ▐██████████

Date: April 22, 2011

Subject: Production of the antigen and antibody of pancreatic
cancer RIP1

Dear Mr. Andraka,

I regret to inform you that your sensor proposed in the attached procedure would in no capacity perform its intended function. The idea of a carbon nanotube transistor would require such a massive amount of resources that the end product would be prohibitively expensive, incredibly delicate, and low in sensitivity and selectivity. Please consider trying a different approach.

Sincerely,

▐██████████████████

My parents were sitting across from me on the sofa, and they were not happy.

"Jack, don't you think this idea is just a little far-fetched?"

My father was wearing that worried look—again. His eyebrows arched, his hand touching his chin.

My mother was sitting next to him. She stared straight ahead, arms folded across her chest, studying me intently. My parents had recently been forced to do some reassessing since my guidance counselor called. I've learned that guidance counselors tend to call home when students have tried to commit suicide in a bathroom stall.

"We just don't want to see you get hurt, Jack," she said.

She thinks I can't take the pressure.

"You gave it a great try. Maybe it's time to turn the page. Or set

$$C_6H_8O_7 + 3NaHCO_3 \rightarrow 3CO_2 + 3H_2O + 3Na^+ + C_6H_5O_7^{3-}$$

your sights on a different goal," she added.

A different goal? Give up?

I had invested too much time and fought too hard. And I was so . . . very . . . close.

It was clear how uncomfortable this whole experience was for my parents. I could see it in their eyes and their posture. They felt obligated to give me a reality check.

But I felt obligated to ignore it. In fact, I was no longer listening. I had zoned out. At this point, I could practically predict what they would say next, because I had already heard all these arguments in my own head a thousand times over.

The arguments went something like this: Who did I think I was? Did I really think that I knew better than all these PhD expert types? Did I really think that my idea would work?

"No matter how much you believe in your idea, we all know it can't happen without someone willing to let you test it out in an actual laboratory, Jack."

I felt exhausted. I couldn't remember the last time I had gotten a full night of sleep. For months I had been running on nothing but adrenaline. I began to wonder if this was what it felt like to crash.

"If you'd discovered a new way to detect pancreatic cancer, don't you think that one of the doctors would have given you a chance?"

Almost two hundred scientists. Not one thought my idea was credible enough.

What my parents couldn't see, what no one could see, was that in my mind's eye, everything was so clear. A drop of blood on a strip of paper. That was all it would take to test for pancreatic cancer. It was simple, really. If I was right, I was on the brink of a ground-breaking early-detection test with the potential to save millions of people.

None of that mattered, though, if I never made it into a lab.

My parents turned toward each other. They were finally ready to make a decision. They knew how crucially I needed their support. Without it, how was I going to fund my research, or go get the supplies I needed? After all, at the age of fourteen, I wasn't able to drive the family station wagon by myself.

"Okay," my mom finally said. "Let's see where this goes."

It wasn't exactly a ringing endorsement, but it was all I needed.

My uncle had died. I had faced years of bullying and depression. This was what I had. I was not about to give up now.

Not when I was so close.

My test works. I know it does. I just have to prove it to the rest of the world. I just need that one chance.

Chapter 1
GROWING UP ANDRAKA

I was born into a house that looked, from the outside, like the other houses on our block in suburban Maryland. But inside, our house was bursting with creative energy. My parents believed that life was a giant puzzle, and we had the happy task of discovering its infinite mysteries.

For my third birthday, my parents gave me a six-foot-long plastic model river, complete with running water. My father, Steve, who works as a civil engineer, thought it would be fun and educational. I spent hours dropping pieces of foam and other objects into my little river. Using different-sized rocks, I watched, utterly transfixed, all the ways obstructions would change the flow of the water. My very first science experiment was a huge success—banana peels sink.

When I was growing up, my mom, Jane, could turn even a boring car ride into an intense, brain-racking competition between my brother, Luke, and me. In most cases, the challenge began with an innocent question tossed out by my mom.

"What would happen if the sun disappeared? Go!" Mom asked.

Game on. From the backseat, my brother and I raced each other for the right answer.

"The earth would shoot off its orbit!" he shouted.

"It would get really cold," I added.

As fast as my brain worked, Luke's moved even faster.

"We wouldn't know about the sun disappearing for a full eight minutes because of the time it takes for light to travel."

He was so smart and he knew it. Show-off.

"That's not true," I protested.

"Look it up," he said calmly, appearing way too satisfied. We both knew he was correct. He had an annoying habit of always being right.

After my mom felt like our brains had been thoroughly exhausted by one type of question (or, in my case, if she suspected I was on the verge of throwing one of my I'm-tired-of-playing-this-game tantrums), she'd abruptly move on to another, sometimes cutting us off mid-sentence.

"Picture an imaginary frog jumping on a number line. The frog always jumps the same number of steps, but we can't tell you the interval. What numbers do you hit to catch the frog? Go!"

Luke and I blurted out different patterns of numbers.

"Zero, three, seven!" Luke shouted.

"One, four, nine!" I chimed in.

We would know who got the right answer by the compliment from my mom that followed, which usually sounded something like "Great job, Luke," followed by an overly exaggerated sigh huffing out of me.

I can't remember a time when I didn't want to be like my big brother. It seemed like anything he set his mind to he could accomplish, especially if it involved computers, video games, math, or building things. Especially building things. Luke, who had a two-year head start on me from birth, had always loved engineering. Even as a kid, he walked around the house with his little Phillips head screwdriver, taking things apart and trying to put them back together. Sometimes he'd disappear outside, only to show up a few hours later with a broken radio that someone had tossed out in the trash.

On Saturday mornings, when most kids were watching cartoons, I woke up to find Luke hiding away in a corner working like a mad scientist. When I toddled my way over to see what he was doing, he looked at me like a mischievous cat that had caught a mouse and was determined to protect his prized catch from outsiders. I knew he didn't want to be disturbed, so I'd plant myself a safe distance away and watch. Watching Luke in action topped cartoons any day.

By the time I was ready for elementary school, Luke had taught me how to play Chinese checkers. I was so competitive and wanted to beat him so badly. In addition to harnessing the concepts of strategy, playing against Luke also gave me an opportunity to test my death glare. I fantasized that my stare could penetrate his skull, blocking his mental powers and handing me my first victory. I played and glared and glared and played, but no matter how hard I squinted, I always lost. After defeat, I glared at him some more. He'd just laugh and pat my shoulder.

"Maybe next time," he'd say. Both of us knew he didn't mean it.

While his cheerful manner just made me angrier, he didn't seem concerned. He was always moving on to his next intellectual conquest.

On rainy days, my brother and I fought for control of the family computer. It was a big desktop and I loved watching the letters and numbers I touched on the keyboard show up on the screen in front of me. By the time I was in third grade, I was able to open different programs that allowed me to paint or type stories. It wasn't long after I mastered opening and closing my browser that my uncle Ted first turned me on to the powers of the internet.

"Use your technology," he always said. "It goes well with your brain."

He was right. It did. I couldn't believe the wealth of information inside that machine. To eight-year-old me, it seemed like I could discover the entire knowledge of the universe if I hit the right keys.

My uncle Ted and I had a special connection. Actually, Ted wasn't even my real uncle, but since I had never known life without him, he was family. Some of my favorite childhood memories are the summer mornings when Uncle Ted picked me up and took me crabbing. The night before a crabbing day felt like Christmas Eve. I'd lay all my clothes out on my dresser and set my alarm a full hour early, checking it and double-checking it to make sure it was set, before climbing into bed. But it didn't matter how early I set my alarm, I always woke up before it. I'd get dressed quickly and stare out my bedroom window, waiting to see the headlights of Uncle Ted's beat-up blue car pull down the driveway.

When he finally arrived, I'd jump into the passenger seat. Uncle Ted was a big, stocky man, and his brown hair almost touched the ceiling of the car.

"Good morning, Jack. You ready?" he asked, smiling.

"Yeah!"

We'd spend the hour-long ride to his crabbing boat planning the most effective way to catch as many crabs as possible, arriving just as the sun began to rise over the Chesapeake.

When Uncle Ted found a good spot in the bay, we took out our crab pots, which are about the size of medium dog cages, and baited them with chicken necks before dropping them into the water.

The next several hours we spent cruising around the water, talking about anything and everything. Especially the future.

"Have you decided what you are going to be when you grow up, Jack?" he asked.

"I'm going to be a doctor," I told him.

"Why?"

"I want to help people get better," I said proudly.

He smiled.

After giving the crabs enough time to crawl into our pots, Uncle Ted looped the boat back to where we dropped the first pot, and I helped him haul them up to the deck. The pots were now dripping and heavy with crabs. Sometimes a little crab would squirm its way to freedom, scurrying across the deck of the boat, and it was my job to track them down. Luckily, I was quicker than the crabs. If they were very small, I threw them back into the water, where they hit the surface with a tiny smack before disappearing in the waves.

There are few feelings more satisfying than the drive back after a hard day's work of trapping crabs. When we got home, Uncle Ted steamed the crabs and I covered the outdoor tables with newspaper. That night our families gathered around to tell stories and eat crabs. We used mallets and little forks to dig out the tender meat until our tables were a mess of crab shells and the smell of steamed seafood. From my perch at the kids' table, I could hear Uncle Ted's booming laugh. Even when I couldn't hear exactly what the adults were saying, the laughter was contagious. I would fall asleep tired and full, listening to the sound of crickets outside my window.

Our house was surrounded by forests. There were trails in every direction, and Luke and I spent our evenings and weekends exploring them, especially the dark and twisty ones. We saw everything from groundhogs and squirrels to snakes. One of the trails led to a creek where Luke and I hunted for salamanders. They liked to hide under the rocks, and we took turns pulling up the rocks and trapping the salamanders in our hands. Their bodies were wet and sticky, with bright spots of color, and we examined them closely, watching the way they squirmed and how the light reflected off their skin, before releasing them. After a long day of exploring, we would arrive home to find warm macaroni and cheese waiting for us. We quickly discovered that macaroni and cheese from a box was all that my dad knew how to make.

My mom was often away when I was in elementary school. Our town of Crownsville, Maryland, is just outside Annapolis, and about an hour north of Washington, DC, but my mother did not work nearby. Every Saturday my family piled into our station wagon and drove her to the airport so she could catch a flight to Cleveland, Ohio, where she worked as a nurse anesthetist. Five days later, we'd pick her up.

The idea that my mom was a sleep doctor fascinated me. As soon as I was old enough to talk, I began begging her to let me fly to Ohio to watch her in action. I wanted to see a real-life surgery in the worst way. I had spent hours online pulling up videos of surgeries.

Watching doctors open up people was even more interesting than watching Luke open up radios. I wasn't grossed out by it at all. However, when my mom finally did decide to let me and Luke fly along with her to Cleveland, it wasn't for a field trip to the hospital. Instead, she dropped us off for a week at a farm. Seriously. "Kids love farms," my mom said as she waved good-bye. "You will have a great time!"

I had a terrible time. My brother and I worked these crazy twelve-hour days shoveling cow poop while trying not to freeze to death or get buried in the six-foot-high snowdrifts. I had never wanted to get back to Crownsville so badly. At least I knew I wasn't going to be a farmer when I grew up.

The next year, when my mom took a job in Washington, DC, I was ecstatic. It wasn't only because the closer commute meant more time together. More important, now that her work didn't involve airplane tickets, it meant I would finally be able to watch a real-life surgery!

I was in second grade when the big day came. I got all dressed up in green scrubs and washed my hands with special soap. The surgery was a simple procedure. A doctor was removing a clot from someone's foot. My mom's role in the whole process seemed anticlimactic. She basically stood watching a sleep-medicine machine, which wasn't all that exciting. What did amaze me was the skill and precision of the doctors around the operating table. The entire surgery lasted only forty minutes, but I was transfixed for each second.

The doctors looked so calm as they cut into that person's foot.

The more I learned about surgeries on the internet, the more my mom's job became an endless source of fascination. I sat cross-legged in my footy pajamas, listening to her talk about her work, and it was better than story time! She explained the chemistry of how the different elements of the anesthesia integrated with the body to make people fall into a kind of deep sleep where they didn't feel the doctors' knives cutting their internal organs. It was hard for me to grasp—I was sure that I would feel it! It also inspired a great sense of wonder. I asked question after question.

Some of the most interesting stories my mom had were about the people she had met. My favorite was the one about the very, very large lady who showed up at the hospital with chest pains. The doctors decided that they needed to put her in surgery, and everything was going as expected, until the moment when the procedure had been completed and the woman woke up. The staff saw her inexplicably digging her hand deep beneath one of her flabs of flesh. When her hand reemerged seconds later, she was clutching a Twinkie. The horrified medical team stopped what they were doing and stood in awe as the lady stuffed the Twinkie into her mouth. The staff later learned it was a game she and her husband played where they hid sweet treats in different parts of their bodies. Her explanation to the doctors was simple enough: she had woken up hungry from surgery, so why not?

* * *

It didn't take long for Mom to begin implementing her core parenting philosophy that kids should be signed up for every activity under the sun, then be allowed to choose what they like.

"Life is all about finding your passion, Jack," my mom was fond of saying. It led to a lot of experiences—and failures.

It began when my parents bought a piano for Luke and paid a conservatory-trained Russian lady to come to our house and give him lessons. I decided to give it a try. To my delight, it appeared to be the one thing my perfect sibling couldn't master, and the more he hated the piano, the more I liked it. The thing I liked best was the thought of beating my brother at something. The moment Luke announced he was quitting piano, I stepped right up and volunteered to take his place.

At first I loved it. I practiced all the time—although never enough for the conservatory-trained Russian lady—but more than enough to get polite applause from the room full of proud parents at recitals. After a while, though, I realized that since I had proven I was better than my older brother at *something*, much of the excitement I had felt over playing started to fade.

Next, my mom thought it was time to sign me up for sports, which quickly proved to be an epically bad idea. Baseball ended when it became clear that I was far more interested in daydreaming and making daisy chains off in right field than hitting or catching the ball. Tennis, which my mother affectionately referred to as a "life-time sport," was even worse. It was scorching hot, and all the other kids had already had years of lessons and were much better. The ground was made of sand or hard dirt, so there weren't even any daisies to make chains with. If the goal was getting my face smashed by the tennis balls, then I would have been closing in on winning Wimbledon by now. Lacrosse, which was also my mother's idea, was almost as bad as tennis. My mother figured lacrosse would be a good choice, mostly because I could use Luke's old equipment. I spent most of lacrosse camp scarring my coaches by singing off-key into my lacrosse stick and trying to avoid getting knocked down.

The only sports I seemed to like were kayaking and white-water rafting. I had always been fascinated by the water. My parents had met on the river, so perhaps it was simply in my blood. On the weekends, my family often went to Pennsylvania or West Virginia,

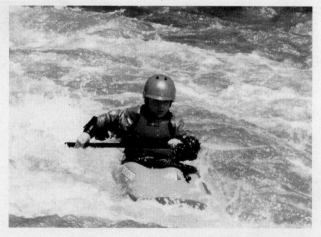

Learning how to kayak on the Nantahala River

where my parents dropped us off so they could kayak the Cheat, Youghiogheny, or Gauley rivers. After they finished, they picked us up to raft a calmer section.

For me, kayaking was a rush. My favorite spot, the Cheat Canyon, has over two dozen rapids rated at least Class III and even some Class IV and Class V rapids, which are for real experts only. My parents guided me down the easier spots. I felt like an action figure in my bright orange kayak, navigating nature's obstacle course. The river was its own living, breathing organism, with plenty of mood swings. Sometimes, it seemed smooth and calm, and then suddenly the water would pick me up and toss me like a leaf and I would go spinning in a new direction. I stared intently downriver, examining the rapids and trying to find the best path downstream.

Sometimes when the water was too high, I walked along the banks with my dog, Casey, a golden retriever, and threw rocks and sticks in the river. I loved building miniature dams and rapids out of the river rocks. I pretended that small twigs were family members and released them down the "rapids," narrating the results, to my parents' horror.

"There goes Mom over a treacherous waterfall!" I said.

"What about Dad?" she asked.

"Oh, Dad is safe. He made an eddy by the rock and he is going to run the Class V rapid," I answered.

Years later, my mom still holds a grudge because she was the

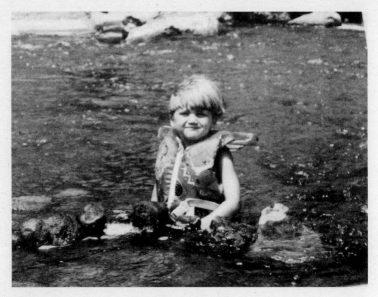

Me building a dam out of rocks

one who always came to the tragic end.

I was the only elementary school kid I knew who was obsessed with low head dams, which are places in a river where the current runs like a giant washing machine. Low head dams are also known as drowning machines because of the way the force of the water can keep swimmers pinned under. There happened to be this huge low head dam right above the campground where we often stayed. I always wanted to take a walk there and, of course, reenact all kinds of drama with twigs and rocks in the river. My mom, again, always met a cruel fate. Maybe she shouldn't have pushed me into tennis!

* * *

It wasn't long before I found another love—this time in math. Searching for subtle patterns and working out problems always made me excited. Not only did I enjoy it, but I was good at it too. Unfortunately, my elementary school didn't teach much math. In fifth grade, we were still learning to tell time!

I learned more about math at home than I did in school. My mom brought me home fun math packets to keep me challenged, but more than anything, it was Uncle Ted who introduced me to a new way of looking at numbers.

Whenever he saw me struggling, he picked up a pencil and offered me help.

"What's the problem?" he asked.

"Everything," I replied.

His mind worked like a beautiful machine that connected everything into understandable patterns. By using visualization techniques, he could make my math problems leap off the page and come to life.

"Here, watch, I have a little trick to show you," he said. "Give me seven numbers. Any numbers. It doesn't matter which ones."

I spouted out the first seven random numbers that came to mind. I watched as he picked up the pencil and began furiously scribbling.

I couldn't believe my eyes. In under ten seconds, after writing down just a few numbers, he had divided a six-digit number by nine. It couldn't be possible.

"No way!" I said.

"Check me."

I punched the numbers into my calculator.

"It's right," I said in disbelief. "How did you . . ."

He looked down at me, smiling. It was the kind of smile that revealed he had a secret to share.

"Let me show you how," he said.

He walked me through a process I never knew existed of making calculations mostly in my head. It was a superfast long-division trick that stayed with me. It was also my first introduction to mental math. Uncle Ted taught me math shortcuts; by estimating and quickly using math facts that are committed to memory, such as multiplication or division, I learned how to solve problems faster.

From that point forward, I began to see patterns in everything I did. With math, I no longer thought of what I was doing as educational or anything remotely associated with work, or school. I just thought of it as solving the mysteries of the universe. Some nights I hid under my covers studying math problems with a flashlight when I was supposed to be sleeping.

My newfound passion for math snowballed into the revelation that there was something else I enjoyed and seemed naturally good at—science.

I had always liked doing experiments. I started with basic ones like working out how many books I could rest on eggs before they cracked, or making water boil at different temperatures using salt. By the time I entered fifth grade, my experimentation began to take on a life of its own. One day I decided to cultivate E. coli, a bacteria that can cause deadly infections, just for the fun of it—on the kitchen stove. That was the last day of science experiments in the kitchen. From that point on, my parents insisted that I use the basement as my lab.

In the darkness of the basement, I labored on an experiment in one corner while my brother, Luke, worked on much more serious experiments in the other. I didn't always know what he was doing, but I knew enough to be afraid. Sometimes, very afraid.

My brother and I were always pushing it. One day Luke had taken apart an old microwave he had found in someone's garbage and was making a ray gun that he was using to roast things. I was on the other side of the basement trying not to get too freaked out by what my brother was doing while I experimented with capacitors, which are like little sponges that quickly soak up electricity. I wanted to see what would happen if I supercharged some particles to create plasmas with aluminum foil.

That's when everything in the basement went black.

"We must have blown a fuse," Luke said.

We didn't realize it, but we were using way too much energy. Our parents weren't home, so Luke walked to check the fuse box. A few minutes later, we heard a knock on the door. It was the power company. We hadn't just knocked out the power to our own house. We had knocked out the power for the whole neighborhood! Whoops.

"Did either of you notice anything unusual?" the worker asked, looking suspiciously around the house.

Luke and I looked at each other nervously.

"No, sir," I muttered.

There was nothing unusual, I told myself to justify the lie. In the Andraka house, at least, this was a normal afternoon.

When my parents got home from work that night we fessed up. Instead of getting angry and grounding us like we had expected, Mom and Dad looked both terrified and amused as they pleaded with us to be more careful and not blow the house up. Dad ended his speech with a warning.

"You are not to talk about what happened," he said. "Ever." (Sorry, Dad!)

My parents often found themselves in a difficult position. They didn't want anyone to get hurt, but at the same time, they felt it was important to let me and Luke experiment and learn on our own terms. And it was working. My mind was growing in ways I never knew were possible, and my parents had taken notice. When it became clear my elementary school wasn't challenging me, my mom went out and found a small charter school nearby that specialized in math and science, where I could progress at my own pace.

The difference between my charter school and my public school was like night and day. The first thing I realized about my new school when I started sixth grade was that the students were hypercompetitive, especially when it came to the mandatory Hunger Games–style contest called the Anne Arundel County Regional Science and Engineering Fair.

Much like the actual Hunger Games, this contest was a complete bloodbath. Once a year, the entire student body assembled at the University of Maryland to duke it out, project versus project. The last student standing would receive bragging rights over the entire school, along with a cheap laptop. Every time I thought about winning the contest, I felt a shot of adrenaline. I love competition. I was all in.

The beginning of sixth grade was also when I met Logan.

I was sitting in Advanced Math class when I first laid eyes on her. She and I hit it off right away. Each time the teacher had his head turned to the board, we passed notes back and forth.

"Want to sit next to me at lunch?" I wrote.

"Yes," she'd write back.

It didn't take long for the relationship to evolve out of the classroom. We spent as much time as possible hanging out. We had a natural, easy connection. Before long, people assumed we were an item, and we were both happy to go along with it.

"I guess we are boyfriend and girlfriend," I said.

"Cool," she answered.

That was that. My first girlfriend.

As a present, she bought me a stuffed brown bear and chocolates. Now that I was in middle school, I was beginning to notice the pressure to fit in. Being with Logan made me feel normal and accepted. And she was the perfect girl—beautiful, smart, and, above all else, fun to be around.

Our favorite thing to do was go to the movies together, then go back to her house, where we had noodle fights in her gigantic pool. We couldn't stop laughing. Everything was funny to us. It all seemed perfect.

A few weeks into our relationship, however, I began to feel that something was very wrong. I loved spending time with Logan. I liked the smiley faces she wrote on the notes that we passed back and forth in class and sitting across from her in the cafeteria, hearing her easy laugh. But there was something missing. I was supposed to be feeling something for Logan that I wasn't sure I was feeling. Specifically, I was supposed to want to kiss her. And the truth is . . . I didn't. After the first month of sixth grade had gone by without me making a move for that first kiss, I knew that Logan was beginning to wonder what was up too.

For the first time, a new question began swirling around my head, and this one had nothing to do with polynomials or water-saturation levels or choosing an extracurricular activity.

What is wrong with me?

$C_6H_8O_7 + 3NaHCO_3 \rightarrow 3CO_2 + 3H_2O + 3Na^+ + C_6H_5O_7^{3-}$

Chapter 2
THE GEEK IN THE CLOSET

As sixth grade progressed, I still wasn't feeling anything for Logan. I was very confused.

The question was always there.

She's perfect. Why aren't I attracted to her?

Fortunately, Logan hadn't brought it up. That was a relief.

I did everything I could to push thoughts like that to the furthest and darkest corners of my mind. I told myself that everything was great. And besides my confusion over Logan, my year was going well. I had made two new friends, Jake and Sam, and the three of us were inseparable. Jake was the kind of guy who would do almost anything if you dared him to. He had so much energy that he made me and Sam laugh all the time. Sam was a little calmer. He had a great sense of humor and was the kind of friend who was simply easy to be around. On the weekends we had sleepovers together and stayed up all night playing World of Warcraft, listening intently to make sure that our unsuspecting parents didn't find out. Sometimes we'd take trips to Hershey Park to ride the roller coasters and eat junk food. More often than not, we made our own fun. Jake had a huge trampoline in his backyard, and we'd throw a black ball onto the top and all try to jump without touching the ball. Exhausted and sweaty, lying on my back on the trampoline, I didn't want to confront my confusion or think about serious things. I just wanted to have fun.

One day, I was sitting with Jake, Sam, and Logan for a game of Truth or Dare. My seat was located inside a large cardboard box, the result of a previous dare.

We were waiting to see who Jake would pick next. He turned to me.

"Jack," he said. "Truth or dare?"

Everyone knows I always pick dare. I'm just that kind of guy.

"Dare."

Jake flashed a mischievous smile.

"Kiss Logan," he said.

"What?" I answered, even though I'd heard him perfectly.

"Kiss your *girlfriend*," he said.

"Get some!" Sam said.

What Sam and Jake didn't know was that despite the fact that we had been going out for three months, Logan and I had never kissed.

Not so much as a peck. Now everyone was looking. I felt myself blush. All I wanted to do was disappear inside my box. Maybe seal it with a postage stamp and mail it to some other place.

"No problem," I said. I tried to look confident as I lifted myself out of the box and strode over to Logan.

She could totally sense my nerves, which made her uncomfortable too. She squirmed in her seat. I just wanted to get it over with.

Act natural, Jack. Just act natural.

I planted a long, unnatural peck on her lips, acting like it was no big deal, before retreating back to my box.

She smiled awkwardly. I smiled awkwardly.

"Truth or dare?" I asked Jake, attempting to move the attention on to someone else, anyone else, as quickly as humanly possible.

Oh God. What's going on with me?

Inside, I knew something was wrong. By this age, I had seen enough television shows to know that this experience—my first kiss—should have felt different. I should have been feeling nervous, of course, but mixed with that anxiety should have been a measure of excitement and attraction. However, it didn't feel like I was kissing my girlfriend. Instead, it felt like I was kissing my best friend. My best friend who I wasn't attracted to.

All the thoughts whirling through my head just made me irritable every time I saw Logan.

What's wrong with me?

Why don't I feel that way about her?

Not knowing where else to turn, I began to take it out on Logan. I began hanging out with her less and ignoring her. Eventually my confusion turned into anger. I stopped ignoring her and started acting like I was too good for her. I was a real jerk. Finally, about midway through sixth grade, I sent her a note telling her we were over. Breaking up via note is an amateur move even by an eleven-year-old's standards. It's no surprise that she stopped talking to me.

The self-inflicted loss of Logan didn't completely spell the end of my social life. I still hung out with Jake and Sam, but they had begun to notice some changes in me too. They could tell something was wrong. Sometimes my answers were curt or I seemed distracted. I could feel myself slowly beginning to pull away from them too.

Although my ability to maintain my friendships was breaking down, my competitive spirit began to rev up. The big science fair was coming. I still needed to find an idea for a project, and fast. It wasn't only about bragging rights; it was also a huge part of my final grade.

Inspiration struck while kayaking the Cheat River with Uncle Ted. We came upon a low head dam. However, this time, instead of tossing in sticks to symbolize my various family members, I wanted to understand why it did what it did. I asked Uncle Ted.

"It's known as a submerged hydraulic jump," he said. "It's really fascinating."

As we continued drifting down the Cheat, he began to explain how the dangerous backwash below the dam could be deadly. On the surface, the water looked peaceful, but underneath it was violent and powerful. Anything caught by the backwash could be trapped and recirculated around and around, making escape or rescue difficult or even impossible.

I wanted to learn more. As soon as I got home, I hit the family computer and began to research on the internet. The more I learned, the more I became mesmerized by the laundry machine–like effect of the water, and its ability to hold people down.

I was able to discover that there were thousands of these hidden hazard spots scattered all over the country. It seemed like a year didn't go by without someone drowning from the force of these strange and powerful currents lurking just beneath the surface. I wanted to know everything, especially about the science behind how these drowning-machine dams worked and exactly what was happening under the water.

I began to think, what if I could find a way to change the flow of the water so that it wouldn't pull swimmers down? Then another thought occurred to me—this would be my project. It allowed me to take my fascination with low head dams and turn it into a science fair entry that could help save lives. I took the model river that my dad had helped me make in my basement and began tinkering around and adjusting the water flow to try to replicate what was taking place at the dam. Using all the different case studies, I was able to create an accurate scale model of the river, the low head dam, and a human. I attached a sump pump to the model that allowed me to adjust the flow of my basement river to replicate the flow of the real river. Once I had my model river and model human down to the exact scale to replicate the effect of the drowning machine, I switched out the wooden bottom with a piece of clear Plexiglas that allowed me to monitor the conditions from all vantage points.

Now that I had succeeded in replicating the drowning machine, I needed to find a way to stop the dangerous washing machine–like effect. I spent huge chunks of time in my dark basement experimenting with how different obstructions would alter the flow of the water.

I tested various custom-made pieces of plastic, wood, and concrete. I tried forty different fixtures before finally finding one that could alter the intense cyclical effect of the water. The one I found that worked was a piece of curved wood with a five-to-one slope. By positioning the apex or top of the curve at the center of the dam, the tailwater gradually increases, disrupting the flow of water enough to kick out whoever is trapped. Mission accomplished: the retrofit eliminated the submerged hydraulic jump.

Through replicating a low head dam on a miniature scale, and a process of trial and error, I had solved a problem that was killing people. My experiment successfully proved there was a way to make these low head dams much safer. For the first time in my life, I realized I had the power to make real change in the world.

I couldn't wait to share my idea with my classmates! However, I knew it was a risky move. Revealing details about science projects was just not something a lot of people did at this school. Remember when I referred to the science fair as the Hunger Games? Well, that was only a slight exaggeration. The competition really was ruthless, and there were rumors that students weren't above sabotage. I believed them.

The one person I would have felt comfortable telling was Logan, but I had completely screwed that up. She still wasn't speaking to me. But I couldn't help myself. I just had to tell someone. I was talking to Jake before class when I decided I couldn't contain my excitement for another second.

Jake had just the reaction I'd been hoping for. The more he heard, the more impressed he sounded.

"Seriously, you have a great chance of winning," he said.

"Really? You think?"

The idea of actually winning the science fair wasn't something that had entered my mind. My only real expectation was to get a good grade.

"No, really, Jack, your idea is awesome," he added. I could tell he meant it.

As Jake asked more and more questions about my project, I was so excited to share my ideas with him that I began to speak louder. A boy named Damien overheard me.

I've come to believe that there is at least one kid like Damien in every school. Damien was simply a jerk. A huge jerk. He always had a problem with me. I could tell he was supercompetitive like everyone else, but for whatever reason, he hated me in particular. That was the only way I could think to explain his behavior. Like randomly walking over to me to tell me how much I sucked. Damien was overly fond of the word *suck*.

"You're doing your project on low head dams?" he asked with a smirk. We both knew it wasn't really a question. It was a taunt.

I just didn't want to deal with him. Not now. Not ever.

"Maybe, why?" I answered, turning away.

"Well, it sounds like your project really sucks," he said.

There it was. His favorite word—*sucks*.

"I'm going to win," he added, that smirk back on his face. "But I'm just kidding, I'm sure you'll do great."

I wasn't very good at these kinds of conversations where what is being said is very different from what is meant.

"Well . . ." I sputtered.

I was racing to think of a comeback, but my mind blanked.

Luckily, that was the moment when our teacher showed up and unlocked the classroom door, saving me from looking like an idiot. I took my seat and began fuming. Damien had always annoyed me, but this time he really struck a nerve.

This kid doesn't even know me! Why does he think he's all that?

I wanted to beat him. Badly.

If I really was going to have a chance to crush Damien, I knew I needed to get to work, and fast. There were only seven weeks until the fair. I knew my science was solid, but I wasn't so sure about my speaking and delivery, which were almost as important as the project in these competitions.

I rehearsed over and over in front of my parents. My first clue that something was wrong came from the look of boredom that spread across their faces as I was giving my presentation. After a few rehearsals, my parents decided they were done hearing me practice my talks. They bought me a video camera and told me to watch myself. Talk about a rude awakening! All along, I had thought I was doing okay while delivering speeches, but when I watched myself on the video, I realized I wasn't just bad—I was horrible.

I gulped. I stuttered. I lost where I was on my board and droned on and on. I had to start over every time I made a mistake.

Needing help, I sunk to a level no little sibling should ever sink to—I asked my older brother for advice. After watching me go through the motions of my presentation, he responded in the only way he knew how.

"You stink," he told me, and shut the door in my face.

He came back a little later and shoved a piece of paper at me. "Here's a card with tips I've learned that I wrote down for you," he said. "Now quit bothering me until you learn them."

I devoted hours to studying those cards, which had useful tips
like:

"Talk like you are telling a friend about a new game where you
know all the info, but it's still a conversation."

"Say what you think, don't give a speech."

"Never go back! Keep moving and incorporate missed parts
later."

"Keep it neat."

"Lose all the boring stuff."

I studied YouTube videos of science fair presentations, and practiced more and worked more.

Slowly, I began to see results. My delivery got smoother. The
more I practiced, the more confident I became. The more confident I became, the less I gulped or stuttered. As the date of the fair
approached, I finally felt ready.

On the day of the competition, I arrived at the University of
Maryland hoping to get a great grade, best Damien, and maybe
even place somewhere in one of the eight different categories. The
categories ranged from chemistry to engineering to physics. After
all the special category winners are announced, the judges award
the second and first runners-up before crowning the fair's ultimate
champion.

After pushing through the wide double doors, I felt like I was
walking right into one of the YouTube clips I had studied. There were

booths set up all over a large convention floor and clusters of kids swaying nervously back and forth in front of their projects. I didn't do a lot of talking. I had my game face on, which looks a lot like my regular face except I'm not smiling.

I found my spot and finished setting up my display, a large piece of cardboard with "Can We Stop the Drowning Machine?" written on top, along with information on how I reached my conclusions. Then it was time to scope out my competition. I didn't think I had much of a shot at winning since it was my first real science competition and there were so many really great projects, especially from the seventh and eighth graders. In the behavioral science category, one was called "Which Common Beverage Is Most Damaging to Teeth?" In the same category, there was another neat-looking project that had mice running through a maze, called "The Effect of Classical Music on Mice Going Through a Maze." One of my favorites was called

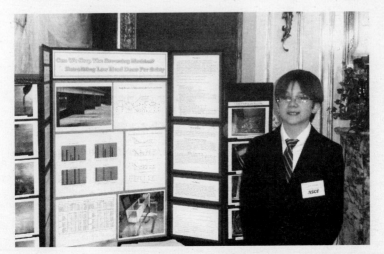

My sixth-grade science fair presentation,
"Can We Stop the Drowning Machine?"

"Maglev Train Speed Efficiency." It featured a Lego train that used magnets to levitate.

Then—I found Damien. He was standing in front of his display, looking smug.

"Hey, loser," he said. "Want to see a demonstration?"

"No thanks," I said, acting disinterested.

My brother, Luke, who was an eighth grader, also entered the contest with his "Is There Fungus Among Us?" experiment. Luke's project demonstrated how fungus that attaches itself to a root can actually help the plant grow.

My experience at the fair took a dramatic turn for the worse after Damien won first place in one of the categories.

Great, I'll be hearing about that for the rest of the year.

At the end of the ceremony, it was time to call out the overall winners. The first name they called was Luke's! He had won third place! I felt so proud of him as I watched him climb the stairs. Then came the announcement for second place, which went to a project called "What Is the Most Efficient Blade Angle for a Windmill?" I loved that project and thought it would win first.

What's going to top that?

You could have heard a pin drop in the auditorium the moment before the judges announced the overall winner.

"And first place goes to Jack Andraka, with his 'Can We Stop the Drowning Machine? Retrofitting Low Head Dams for Safety.'"

My jaw dropped to the ground. From my spot on the stage, I looked out into the audience. I saw my brother smiling. Damien was scampering for the exit.

After hugging my mom and dad, I couldn't wait to call Uncle Ted and tell him the news. I grabbed my mom's flip phone.

"Uncle Ted, guess what?" I said.

"What? How did you do?"

"I won," I said.

"That's great. Which category?"

"The whole thing. First place overall!"

He was blown away.

"Congrats, Jack! That's amazing," he said. "We need to celebrate!"

As a reward, he took me on his boat for a day of sailing around on the Chesapeake. I thought that was even better than the laptop the school awarded me for winning. I brought Jake and Sam along with me and made it a party. It was a beautiful day. As we cruised all around the bay, we waved to other boats passing by while we took turns steering.

I'd be back on the boat before long. As sixth grade came to a triumphant end, crab season was just beginning. Even though I was older, I still set my alarm and stared out the window, feeling the same childlike excitement when I saw Uncle Ted's beat-up car will itself down my driveway.

However, this year, I noticed that something was different. As we went through our familiar routine of dumping and pulling up the traps, instead of an abundance of crabs, there were only a handful.

"What's happening?" I asked. "Where are all the crabs?"

"The crabs are dying because there is more pollution in the water," he said.

"Why?" I asked.

One of Uncle Ted's favorite topics of conversation was the water quality in the Chesapeake Bay. In his job as a water-quality special-ist, he knew firsthand the devastating effect pollution could have on the fragile marine life and talked for hours about what could be done to prevent it.

"The pollution comes from a lot of different places," he said. "There is a new industrial plant in Baltimore, and I think some of it comes from that. A lot of it is just runoff from people's houses."

I still didn't understand and wanted to know more.

"When people put a lot of fertilizer in their yards to make their grass green and their flowers grow, the runoff goes into the water and makes algae grow in the bay," he said.

I was confused. I thought algae was good.

"How does algae kill crabs?" I asked.

Even though I was just a kid, he spoke to me about his ideas like I was his equal. He just assumed I understood what he was saying, knowing that I would ask questions if I didn't. I always thought that must have been one of the reasons his words stuck to the insides of my brain like they did.

"The algae can block out the sunlight and sometimes leave the oxygen level too low to support marine life like crabs," he said.

It was the first time I had ever considered the problem, and I was fascinated. I began to connect all these different thoughts in my head: the pollution in the Chesapeake Bay has a chain reaction that extended way beyond the water, into almost every aspect of the surrounding ecosystem. As he explained, I could see his words turn into pictures. The pollution that soaks into the water. The fish that soak in the pollution. The people that eat the fish. He ended his story about pollution the same way he ended all his stories, by shaking his head and adding—"There has to be a better way."

We were eventually able to gather enough crabs for our annual crabbing feast. I was looking forward to the rest of summer vacation when my mom had another bright idea: flying me to Colorado Springs to attend a math camp.

I was skeptical that this was a worthwhile investment of my precious summer vacation. A math camp? I mean, it was literally called math camp.

The first day of camp felt like the first day at a new school. A lot of the kids knew each other because they had gone the previous year. I didn't know anyone. On the bus ride that took us from the airport to the camp site, I sat quietly by myself.

That's when an older girl came up to me and introduced herself.

"Hi, I'm Katherine, where are you from?"

"Maryland," I replied meekly.

Katherine took me under her wing immediately. She was an eighth grader and she acted like a big sister. I'd never had a big sister before, and I liked how she showed me around and introduced me to the people she knew.

Not only did I make a great friend, but I was wrong about the camp. It was so much more than math. Imagine an extended thirty-day sleepover with a group of really cool people. We played lots of card games and watched movies. Even the sports there were fun; we had intense Ultimate Frisbee and soccer matches. In the evenings we played round after round of Truth or Dare. Despite my awkward experience with Logan at the beginning of the year, I remained a dare guy. I also learned how to do origami. Folding paper into intricate shapes became a great way for me to relax and allow my ideas to come to me. At the end of each camp day, Katherine and I found a large sofa in the recreation room, where the big television was, and we curled up and watched *America's Next Top Model* together.

When we did focus on math, it was challenge after challenge. The other campers were smart, and often we became embroiled in mathematical discussions during lectures or in breakout sections about the problems we were solving. We debated about whether math was created or discovered, shared tricks for solving complex

equations, and examined different approaches to the same problems. I was actually sad when camp ended, and I decided I wanted
to go back next year.

After returning home, I discovered two furry additions had been
made to the Andraka family. My mom had surprised Luke and me
with our very own ferrets. I named mine Ginny Weasley, after the
Harry Potter character, and Luke named his Phaedrus, after the
ancient Greek philosopher who once said, "Things are not always as
they seem; the first appearance deceives many." Ferrets make great
pets. They are affectionate and smart, and they sleep all the time.
Ginny Weasley loved to curl up on my shoulder and take a nap as I
read.

They didn't bother Casey, our golden retriever. They arched their
backs and hopped around, goading him to play. Casey stared at them
in amusement but generally didn't pay much attention.

I spent what was left of the summer in my basement working on
more experiments. The more time I spent in the basement, the more
complex my experiments became.

One day, I ordered a bunch of organic molecules including nitrogen off the internet so I could produce a catalyst for breaking down
organic chemicals. It was the first time I started doping titanium
dioxide with nitrogen groups. I just wanted to see what would happen. What I didn't realize at the time was that some of the chemicals I
was buying were also used to make extremely dangerous explosives.

The FBI somehow had access to my purchase history and sent a curt letter to my house letting me know that I was being watched. My mom and dad were not amused. Not even a little. I couldn't help but notice that from that point forward they began to stay farther and farther away from the basement.

Sometimes the experiments I intended to create at the beginning turned into ones I didn't expect. One night I was up late mixing nanoparticles in a breakfast bowl in my kitchen. When I got tired, I went to bed, leaving the bowl out on the counter. The next morning, I woke up and saw my twelve-year-old cousin Allen in the kitchen.

"Hey, I forgot you were coming," I said.

He looked up and waved, too busy to give a proper greeting, since he was plowing spoonfuls of cereal into his mouth. I noticed something familiar about his bowl. My morning brain slowly made the connection.

My experiment!

I looked around the counter for my nanoparticles. They were gone. I looked back at my cousin. He had poured his milk and cereal into my experiment bowl and was slurping up the nanoparticles, which look like white powdery sugar.

"Dude, stop eating that!" I yelled.

He looked up, nanoparticle-infused milk dripping from his mouth.

"You're eating my science experiment!"

He spit out the cereal and ran to the bathroom.

Since that day, I joke around, telling him that he's my walking science experiment and I'm closely monitoring him, chronicling the results each time he visits.

With one week left of vacation before seventh grade, I got terrible news. My two best friends, Jake and Sam, were both moving out of state. It was a rough blow, but I tried to stay positive. After all, making new friends at math camp hadn't been too hard. Plus, I was coming off a first-place victory in my first science fair. That should earn me some new friends, I thought.

However, another, even more disruptive change was going on inside me. When seventh grade started, a lot of the guys at school couldn't help but notice how much the girls had matured over the summer. No matter how hard I had tried to ignore my feelings, it was becoming even more obvious that I wasn't into girls.

One day I found myself daydreaming about a male classmate. *He's cute*, I thought to myself. Sometimes I laughed a little too long at a boy's joke, or spaced out in class, thinking about boys. As seventh grade went on, these feelings and thoughts of attraction were becoming more and more difficult to block out. They were happening all the time.

What is going on with me?

Despite the obvious signs, I wasn't really sure, or ready to confront, what it all meant. I didn't know how people would react, but

I had a sinking feeling it wouldn't be good. I took my feelings and I locked them deep in a vault, and I did my very best to forget about them entirely.

I stayed focused on science. That was something that made complete sense to me. What I love most about science is how it allows me to peek into a different world, taking me to a deeper place, behind the seemingly random colors and shapes all around us, to a reality of rules and principles, a destination where the more I learn and the more layers I pull back, the closer I can come to unlocking the secret behind every problem or mystery in the universe. In science, contradictions don't exist. Every action has a cause and every problem has an answer, if only I can inspire myself enough to find it. I felt like there was no limit to what I could accomplish.

I could tell I was getting better at it too. My confidence was growing. My mind felt like a powerful weapon I could set loose on any problem.

When one of my favorite beaches was closed due to pollution, I saw how local officials had to lug all this expensive equipment to find out what was going on in the water. Not only were the tests expensive, but the equipment wasn't always readily available.

Fresh in my mind was my conversation about crabbing with Uncle Ted and how the pollution in the Chesapeake Bay had killed off so many of the crabs.

There has to be a better way.

Based on everything I had learned studying creeks, I thought I could come up with a solution. I had a feeling that a better indicator of pollution might be found in how bioluminescent organisms, those tiny organisms that emit light, react to contaminants. I began culturing bioluminescent bacteria in the only room in the house that had no windows—the bathroom. After a few weeks, I had so many glowing organisms in there that my mom could read a book without turning the lights on.

By exposing the different organisms to various levels of contaminants, I was able to show that the more pollution the bioluminescent organisms took up, the duller their light became. I had decided to name this year's school project "A Bright Detective: Can Vibrio Fischeri Detect Bioavailable Water Pollutants in the Stony Creek Watershed?" Now that I had a year of experience under my belt, I felt confident that I could have another good showing at my school's science fair, and I did. For the second straight year, I came away with first overall at the Anne Arundel County Regional Science and Engineering Fair.

Two years in a row I had won a major award. In the heavily competitive world of science fairs, I was fast earning a reputation as someone to keep an eye out for.

While I was working on better ways to detect pollution, Luke, who was now a freshman in high school and was still in the science fair game, was also knee-deep in water. His project was genius. It

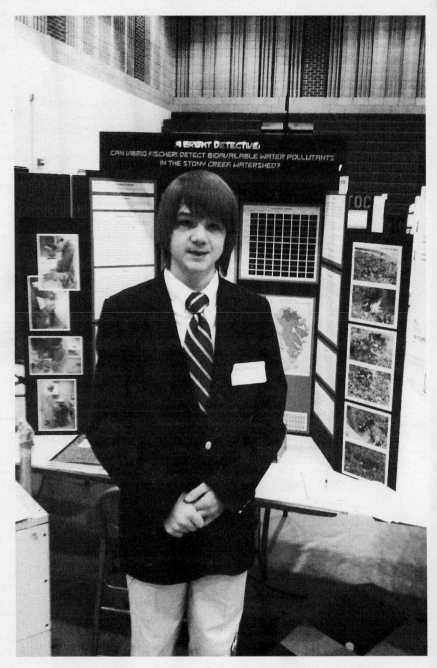

My seventh-grade science fair presentation, "A Bright Detective: Can Vibrio Fischeri Detect Bioavailable Water Pollutants in the Stony Creek Watershed?"

examined acid mine drainage's negative effects on the environment and wildlife and was able to come up with a real-world solution. It was his best project yet.

Luke had designed a cell that allowed him to test four different variables. Given those variables, he was able to create the perfect cell for any stream according to its specific parameters. Not only did it have the potential to change the way we treat the pollution in these streams and save millions of gallons of fresh drinking water, but it was also much easier to implement than the current limestone techniques because his method required less cost and manpower.

Luke titled his project "Electrochemical Remediation of AMD—A Solution to Acid Mine Pollution?"

Luke and I planned to enter our projects into our first non-regional science fair, the International Sustainable World (Energy, Engineering, and Environmental) Project Olympiad (or I-SWEEEP) in Houston, Texas. Now that I had developed the confidence I needed with my public speaking, I thought this time would be easier, but I also knew the competition would be a lot stiffer.

I-SWEEEP was one of the largest environmental science fair competitions in the world, with 1,655 student scientists from 71 countries competing against one another. The stage at I-SWEEEP was bigger than anything I had ever seen in Maryland. And the competition was just unbelievable.

It was my first time at a national award ceremony, and I wasn't focused as much on winning because I didn't think I had a chance. My goal was to soak everything in and hopefully use that knowledge in future projects. It was clear that everything at I-SWEEEP was on a higher level—from the sophistication of the projects to the way the students presented their ideas.

At the fair, I walked the convention hall to check out the other projects, when I saw that a small crowd had gathered around one of the displays. Once I began reading the scientist's board, I was absolutely speechless: she had discovered a new way to detect land mines using sound waves.

I stood there staring in disbelief.

"Hi, I'm Marian Bechtel," the young girl said as she extended her hand to me.

I wanted to know everything. My first question—how?

Marian said she had met a group of international scientists working on a device that used holographic radar to detect buried land mines, and had become inspired by their work. She had been playing the piano when she noticed that the strings on a nearby banjo resonated when she played certain notes or chords. This gave her an idea—she realized that using acoustic or seismic waves to excite a buried land mine could allow for their detection.

"I was able to combine my newfound passion for humanitarian de-mining with my love of music," she said.

Next to her display was a simple prototype of an acoustic

detection device she had created out of the frame of a scrap-metal detector.

Hearing her story made me feel inspired. When it came time to present my idea to the judges, I was on my game. I still had that index card with my brother's tips. I didn't try impressing the judges with big words. Instead, I kept my presentation understandable and interesting.

Like at my local science fair, there were a bunch of different special categories along with an overall winner. I was just happy to be there. When the judges announced that I had finished first place in the nation for middle school, I screamed—not so much out of joy, but out of total shock. It was an unbelievable honor to have my project be recognized nationally in my age group.

However, the biggest news of all was that Luke finished first overall, which meant that he had earned a spot to compete in the Holy Grail of science fairs—the Intel International Science and Engineering Fair (or ISEF).

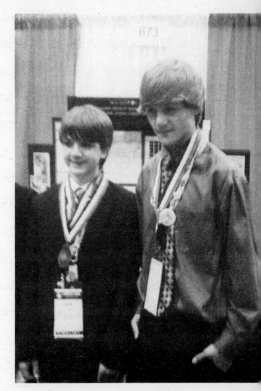

Me and Luke with our I-SWEEEP awards

When my parents told me I was going to accompany him to San Jose, California, where the event was being hosted, I ran around the kitchen island in frantic circles, making everyone, including myself, dizzy.

I arrived at ISEF as his guest and was surprised to see it was nothing like my local science fair, with a mixed assortment of sort-of-good and sort-of-bad projects, or even like I-SWEEEP. ISEF was the best of the best. These kids all had superior projects, and they were passionate, articulate, and brilliant. In a word, they were all perfect.

I got to spend almost a whole week hanging out with these older and wiser kids, and I was totally starstruck. I went up and down the aisles of the science fair like a little kid in a candy shop, asking everyone about their projects. ISEF made these cool cards for each scientist. Each had a picture on one side and a short bio on the back, and I collected the cards of all the finalists and studied them intensely.

How did Luke do at ISEF? Let's just say he won $96,000 in prizes. I'd never felt more in awe of my brother.

The last day of the competition, I was sitting in the audience as Amy Chyao, who was only sixteen years old, walked up to the stage to accept the competition's top prize, the Gordon E. Moore Award, for her amazing experiment that used light energy to activate a drug that kills cancer.

As soon as I returned home to Crownsville, I went online to learn more about Amy Chyao and all the wonderful things she was doing. Her story was even more inspiring than I could have ever imagined.

During her freshman and sophomore years in high school, Amy taught herself chemistry. Then she applied what she had learned to improve photodynamic therapy, the process of treating superficial skin cancers with light. Photodynamic therapy has been around a long time, but it can be used only on cancers that are close to the skin's surface. However, by taking semiconducting nanoparticles, which are just tiny particles that conduct electricity, and exposing them to certain wavelengths of light, Amy figured out that she could generate a form of oxygen that proves deadly to cancer cells. Once these nanoparticles are injected, they travel through the bloodstream or stay localized in tumor sites. The particles Amy developed allow doctors to use targeted light therapy to penetrate even deeper into the body, creating the possibility of treating a wider variety of cancers beneath the skin.

All this from a kid not a whole lot older than I was.

She was brilliant, bold, and, above all, dripping with creativity. All the things that I wanted to be. I began to think to myself—what if I worked really hard? What if I learned and thought like these incredible kids? Maybe one day I could go to ISEF too. Maybe one day I could do something that made a difference in the world like my new hero, Amy Chyao.

I began to daydream about my science future.

* * *

After winning the top prize for middle schoolers at I-SWEEEP, I expected to be greeted like a conquering hero upon my return to school, maybe not by Damien, but by the rest of the students.

I was wrong.

The more my science star was rising, the more I noticed a change in the attitude of a lot of my classmates. At first, I thought it was just in my head. But I began to realize it was a lot more than that. In my hypercompetitive school, resentment over my success was beginning to boil over.

It seemed like overnight everything had changed. When I won an award for the first time in sixth grade, the kids at school seemed happy for me. But now, whenever I spoke about science fairs, I noticed that something seemed to change in the way the other kids looked at me. Instead of sharing in my joy, they seemed angry. I could hear kids whispering about me as I walked down the hall. I could see the smirks and grins out of the corner of my eye.

No matter how many times I told myself I was being paranoid, the evidence kept piling up. During the third week of seventh grade, I walked into the cafeteria, sat my tray down at a table, and watched everyone sitting at the table get up and move. They offered no explanation. They just didn't want to be near me. I felt invisible, like a ghost that people knew was around but didn't want to acknowledge.

Humiliated and wanting to avoid another horrible experience

like that, I decided to skip lunch altogether. After the fourth-period bell rang, I followed all the other kids toward the cafeteria, then at the last second made a beeline straight to the boys' bathroom. There I darted into the handicapped stall, locking the door behind me. Once safely inside, I sat on the toilet lid, unpacked my peanut butter and jelly sandwich, and, using the toilet-paper dispenser as a lunch tray, ate my lunch quickly and quietly. Whenever anyone came to actually use the bathroom, it got particularly uncomfortable. I'd lift my feet up and stop chewing until they had finished their business.

My appearance didn't help. Remember that kid in middle school who had big, thick glasses, wore braces, and was always raising his hand in class? Yeah, that was me. To go along with those character-istics, I also had an unfortunate tendency to get sudden nosebleeds that seemed to happen at the worst-possible times. The small class size was a problem too. Being stuck with the same twenty-four kids for all three years of middle school meant that once you formed your reputation, it was impossible to wash off, no matter how hard you scrubbed.

I thought that changing my style might help. I decided my shaggy hair was so nineties. My mom drove me to our local hair stylist. I asked her for a trendy new look. She gave me a bowl haircut. That haircut earned me the new nickname "Coconut Head." It didn't exactly make sense, considering nothing about my haircut resem-bled a coconut, but my classmates didn't seem to care. Whenever

someone so much as uttered the word *coconut*, laughter always followed.

Jake had moved. Sam had moved. Logan wasn't talking to me.
I was utterly alone. I was also beginning to confront my sexuality.
I couldn't ignore all the signs anymore—I knew I was gay. Still, I
remained determined to at least try to pretend that I was the same
as everyone else. Part of me still held out hope that maybe all these
strange feelings would just go away.

For many reasons, this seemed like the best course of action.
First, there was the built-in gay-hater lingo, which had become an
embedded part of middle school vocabulary. In case you didn't
know, in the kid edition of the dictionary, the word *gay* is a synonym
for weird, uncool, cowardly, or essentially anything that sucks in the
world.

If someone is acting stupid, they are "being totally gay."

If someone lacks courage, they are told, "Dude, stop being gay."

If someone likes the wrong music—yup, you guessed it, that is
"so gay." So as you could imagine, coming out as literally gay didn't
seem like the best option for twelve-year-old Jack.

Even though I had tried to hide it, it was becoming increasingly
clear to everyone at school that I was gay. They now had the perfect
weapon to berate and taunt me.

By the midpoint of my seventh-grade year, it seemed my family
and Uncle Ted were the only ones who still thought I was straight.

Every day after school I came home, took a seat at the kitchen table, and tried to lose myself in the world of math and science. I kept my pain to myself. I still didn't feel comfortable talking about my personal problems, in part because I didn't fully understand them.

It felt like a breath of fresh air when I saw Uncle Ted. He was always so positive. He could tell something was on my mind but didn't want to press me. Instead, he looked down at my paper and shook his head.

"How's it going, Jack?" he asked.

"Well, I'm struggling with square numbers," I said.

"There is a better way," he said as he picked up my pencil. It was another mental math shortcut. This one was even better than the long-division one. Uncle Ted patiently showed me how to work through the problems.

"Jack," he said to me before walking away, "whatever is going on at school, remember that it can be easy to lose yourself, but always try to remember who you are. No one can touch you unless you let them."

It wouldn't be long before his advice was put to the test.

My classmates decided that they needed to bring my differences out into the open. I was waiting along with the rest of my class for my music teacher to come and open the doors, when eight or nine boys surrounded me in a circle.

"What's up, dork?" one kid from the cool clique called out.

Yes, they were talking to me. Of course they were talking to me. I tried to act like I didn't hear it, but that only made the voices louder.

"What are you going to do, loser?"

"Are you going to cry?"

I looked around for the teacher. She was late. The hecklers had an audience and they were prepared to put on a show.

"You know that you aren't going to amount to anything, right, loser?"

It was unprovoked. My only crime was standing outside class quietly. I felt my face turn beet red. I tried to smile. I didn't know what to say, so I didn't say anything.

Where is the teacher!?! Where is the teacher!?!

I lowered my head and waited. I knew the teacher would be there any second. Any second.

The circle tightened.

"Are you going to cry, fag?"

I could now feel the hot breath of their words hitting me. I avoided eye contact. Now I wished I really was invisible. Now I wished there was a hole I could jump into to disappear. Instead the voices kept coming faster and faster.

The teacher will be here any minute. Just hang in there one more minute.

The circle closed in on me. One of the boys pushed me. Hard. I dropped to the floor in one direction. My books flew in another. Of course, that's when my nose started bleeding.

I looked up at my classmates. There was blood on my hands, my books, my clothes, the floor. The whole class was laughing really hard.

"You think you're all that? Look at you now!" I heard one of them taunt as I scurried back to my only safe haven, the handicapped stall in the boys' bathroom. I sat on the seat behind the latched door and cried into my hands. I cried a long time.

After the music class incident, my identity and reputation were officially etched in stone. I was on the Not Cool list, and there was simply nothing I could do to change that. And it wasn't just the students who were against me. Sometimes the teachers and staff joined the chorus of haters. A lot of them were deeply religious, and their worldviews didn't square with my identity. To a lot of them, being gay was wrong and immoral. That meant that the people I was supposed to look up to as authority figures had rejected who I was. They believed that I, *as a person*, was wrong and immoral.

One day when I had gotten something wrong in class, a teacher blurted out, "What are you? Gay?"

It was just four words, but it crushed me.

Is there something wrong with being gay?

Is there something wrong with me?

If there was a hell, I reasoned, it probably looked a lot like my middle school.

* * *

When seventh grade finally came to an end, I felt like letting out one giant exhale.

This year, more than any other, I was looking forward to going crabbing with Uncle Ted.

After we had dropped our traps and drifted out far enough into the water, he asked me about school.

"It's been a little rough," I said, in a comment that could be nominated for the understatement of the year.

I could tell he knew it was more than that.

"Jack, just remember all the things you have to look forward to," he said.

"Middle school can be a rough time, but things will get better in high school. You're going to do great things one day," he said. "I just know it."

The summer before eighth grade also meant my return to math camp. After the wonderful time I'd had the summer before, I couldn't wait to hop on the plane and get as far away from Crownsville as possible. I was looking forward to being myself again.

This year's camp was held in Wyoming, and during the first week, I met a boy named Anthony. He was smart and fun, and he had the same interests that I did. We quickly became great friends, but by the second week of camp, my feelings for him had grown into the more-than-friend territory. I liked him. I was getting the vibe that he liked me too. There was just something about the way he looked at me.

Never had I so enjoyed working on math problems with a partner. We laughed and talked as we raced through the quickest ways to solve problems. There were also these moments, like the one night when we were sitting together on the sofa watching the World Cup, and I could feel that tension building up in the pit of my stomach. I wanted so badly to tell him how I felt. He was accepting and kind, I told myself. It would be safe to be my true self around him.

"Anthony?" I said.

"Yeah?"

Every time I tried, I just couldn't gather my nerves. I was afraid talking about it would mess things up.

"Oh, nothing."

As time went on, I felt an increasing pressure to be honest with him about my feelings. I knew that after math camp was over, there was a chance I'd never see him again. What if my cowardice was jeopardizing what could be the greatest relationship ever?

Finally, on the very last day, I decided—*Screw it, I got this.* The whole camp was playing capture the flag. We were running together when I said, "Stop, there is something I need to tell you."

"What?"

I wanted to tell him everything I had been feeling over the past month. I wanted to be open about who I was, but I couldn't get it out. As the silence grew uncomfortably longer, he began to give me this confused look.

"Yeah?" he said, prompting me to speak.

I knew it was now or never.

"I'm gay," I said.

He looked frozen. Now that I had gotten that out of the way, past the point of no return, I went for the kill.

"And I think you are pretty cute."

"Okay," he said. He took a step back. Then he turned around and ran in the other direction as fast as he could. I crouched down on the ground and covered my face with my hands.

He never spoke to me again.

I spent the flight home bawling my eyes out. No matter what I tried, nothing seemed to work. I began fearing that I had become that kid who spent time in his basement experimenting because there was no one who wanted to be his friend.

Chapter 3

A RECIPE FOR DISASTER

After returning home from math camp, I could feel the pressure building. I didn't want to see anyone. I didn't want to go anywhere. I just wanted to stay in my room.

One day, I heard my mom talking on the phone downstairs, and I decided to sit down in the stairwell to eavesdrop on her end of the call. I couldn't hear much, but I could hear enough to know it was a serious conversation. It was like the barometric pressure had spiked and the air in the room felt all heavy.

It didn't take long before I realized that my mom was talking to someone about my uncle Ted.

He was sick. It was cancer.

Uncle Ted? Cancer?

I took a second to digest the information and thought about what it all meant.

The conclusion I came to was that there was no reason to get emotional or panic.

I didn't know a lot about cancer, but I knew enough to feel sorry for Uncle Ted because he was going to have to go through all kinds of awful treatments, but there was another part of me that kind of shrugged it off.

Lots of people get cancer now, I told myself. *They usually do fine. And this is Uncle Ted! Of course he will do fine!*

After hearing the click of my mom hanging up the phone, I casually walked downstairs and asked her who was on the phone.

"Jack, let's go on a walk," she said.

As we began to walk down the trails by my house, she started opening up. "It's Uncle Ted. He is very sick." She explained that he had pancreatic cancer.

"Is he going to be okay?" I asked.

She hesitated. Her eyes looked strange, as if it was taking a great amount of effort to project calm.

"Uncle Ted has great doctors who are going to do everything they can to make him better," she said.

After the walk, I went to my room, closed the door, buried my head under the covers, and cried. At the time I didn't know why. I told myself I was just tired. After all, I did have a lot on my plate.

Eighth grade was about to begin, and I was dreading going back to school.

I did get one piece of good news before starting school: I received a text from Logan letting me know that she had finally forgiven me for being a jerk to her back in the sixth grade. It wasn't as if we were best friends, but at least we were on friendly terms again. Given my current social standing, I was glad to have someone who didn't hate me.

The first thing you need to understand about my life as I began eighth grade is that there were really two Jacks. First, there was the Jack I let everyone else see. That Jack had life figured out. He was happy. He smiled, won science fairs, got A's in his classes, and even took the trash out without being asked.

That was the Jack I wanted to be. But really I was leading a double life. Beneath the wide smile and first-place trophies, there was another Jack who was profoundly unhappy, and who didn't have any idea what to do about it.

In looking for a solution, my mind kept pulling me back to the world of science. If I could discover the principles behind why I had become an outcast in my school, I was sure I could solve this problem and get my social life back on track. I evaluated the circumstances and came to the conclusion that it wasn't just the way I had treated Logan or my classmates' envy of my science awards. It was deeper than that. It was who I *was* that was the problem.

What can I do?

How can I fit in?

Maybe, if I just kept ignoring the pain, I told myself, everything would magically get better. Note to readers: Be wary of any plan that is dependent on magic.

Making the decision to avoid confronting my feelings meant that all that pain inside me had no release. All those terrible feelings stayed bottled up, and with no outlet, the pressure kept building and building.

I knew that *something* had to change. And it needed to change desperately. I looked at the kids who were popular and how they behaved. Most of them weren't raising their hands all the time or blurting out questions. They got good grades but made a point not to show too much effort. I decided that the first thing I needed to shed was my reputation as someone who loved science and math.

What was cool? Apathy, or not caring about anything, was cool. So I became that guy.

Who cares? Not me. I cared about nothing! Or at least I tried. I *never* let on that I did science and math for fun.

What did I care about?

Video games!

Only nerds try hard in school, right? Let's all play World of Warcraft! And after we're done, let's play it again! Then again . . .

and again . . . and again. If my instructor threw out an equation, I pretended to be clueless. I refused to raise my hand or make eye contact. Whenever the teacher called on me, I shrugged.

However, after a few weeks went by, my classmates were still not accepting me. It became obvious that my apathetic act wasn't going to solve the problem. I decided it was time to reevaluate the situation and try to come up with a new solution.

I know the best way to gain acceptance, I thought. *I'll join them!*

Yes—I joined the chorus of haters.

I began by accepting their language and calling anything that was weird or uncool in the slightest way "gay."

I wore my very best fake smile as I directed the words that had once hurt me so badly at the most susceptible kid I could find. He wasn't hard to find. His name was Andres, and he may have been the one kid in the school who had more trouble fitting in than I did.

Andres was a weird kid. During class he sat in the back of the room all by himself and made these really strange noises. Sometimes he picked his nose and examined it.

Adopting my new persona as a hater, I began my verbal assault by insulting his science fair projects, which was the worst kind of insult at my school.

"Nice project," I said, in a way that let him know I really meant the opposite. Then I attacked his sexuality.

"Don't be gay!"

"That is totally gay!"

"That's gay, gay-gay-gay, GAY!"

I didn't know if he was actually gay or not. It didn't really matter. I felt like a sellout, not only to the kid I was making fun of, but to myself. Just when I thought I couldn't sink any lower, this ultimate act of self-rejection brought me down to a whole new level.

Inside, the negativity kept piling up and the pressure continued building in a vicious circle as my feelings of detachment and isolation began to grow more and more extreme. By midway through eighth grade, the transformation felt complete. That happy young Jack who spent his summers playing with sticks in the river with his family had completely vanished, replaced by a brooding and confused kid with his hoodie pulled up over his head and his hands tucked into his pockets. I could feel the world around me growing smaller and darker.

When I was alone, I cried. When I was in front of other people, I smiled, but I felt like crying—which is way worse than crying alone.

Meanwhile, I went to visit Uncle Ted during his first round of chemotherapy. I had brought a homemade get-well card. I didn't know what to say, and I handed it to him as an icebreaker.

"Thank you," he said.

I sat down on the side of his hospital bed. He looked exactly the same. He still was a big, stocky guy with thinning brown hair just like the last time I had seen him. However, our conversations were now different. Everything felt stilted. He tried to act normal, like nothing was wrong.

"What exactly is pancreatic cancer? When will you be better?"

He didn't want to talk about it and kept changing the subject back to me.

At that moment, nothing was working out for me in my life, and I didn't want to talk about it. Between the two of us, there was not much left to say.

As eighth grade continued, the taunting got worse for me. Every moment I spent in school, I felt as though I were under a microscope. I could never relax, and every time I spoke, it felt as though someone was waiting there to pounce with an insult.

Loser.

Freak.

Jack, you're never going to amount to anything. ANYTHING!

I decided to turn to the one resource that *never* let me down— the internet.

I entered *bullying* into a search engine and found over twenty-five million results.

Unfortunately, not many of them were helpful to me. A lot of the advice on a government-run website that bills itself as a guide for parents to help their children with bullying seemed ridiculously out of touch. There were tips like "Say 'stop' directly and confidently. Stay near adults or groups of other kids." Another site suggested, "Sooner or later, the bully will probably get bored with trying to bother you." There was also "If you're in a situation where you have to deal with a bully and you can't walk away with poise, use humor—it can throw the bully off guard."

Tell them to stop? Tell jokes? Walk away? Stay near adults?

One site even suggested that I "try to talk it out and come to a common place of understanding."

Sure. And then let's all hold hands and sing "Kumbaya."

I began to wonder if maybe a bunch of haters got together to make this website as the ultimate taunt. I noticed that a lot of the advice I found online seemed to push this idea that if only the victim worked a little harder to accommodate the haters, maybe the haters would accept them. Anyone who has actually been through the gauntlet of hate understands that no amount of jokes, walking away, or ignoring can get a hater off your back.

I was fed up with everything. I realized that I wouldn't be able to change *who I was*. See, being gay isn't like having an ugly pair of shoes. I can change my shoes, but my sexuality is part of who I am. When you feel ashamed of who you are as a person, the whole world begins to seem like an alien place where you don't belong. Nothing can feel good. And it didn't. Hiding who I was didn't fool anyone. Joining the chorus of haters proved to be an epically bad idea. Maybe, I thought, if I stopped hiding my sexuality, everything would get better.

I put those awful feelings of rejection from the math camp incident behind me. That was different, I told myself, because I was confessing my feelings about someone else. I thought if I was just honest with everyone about who I was, I'd endure some good-natured ribbing before finally being accepted.

Maybe I was just desperate. I don't know. My memory of those dark days isn't always perfectly clear, but in either case, I had finally made the decision—I was coming out.

I tried to put a positive spin on it. I thought my coming out would be a dramatic and proud moment, like those stories we see on TV or in movies. You know, the ones where the gay kid summons up the courage and makes a heroic stand. Like declaring into the microphone minutes after being declared prom king that, guess what, the prom king is gay, and that's all right because he's really the same guy you just voted for! And then, after a few unsettling moments when all the students nervously look around at one another, a slow, small clap begins to fill the silence—and then, suddenly, that clapping breaks out into frenzied applause until the newly out gay prom king is hoisted off the stage, onto the shoulders of his friends, and triumphantly carried out the door to an upbeat pop song that lets the audience know that only great things lie ahead!

What actually happened wasn't like that.

There was no grand announcement.

There wasn't even an in-person announcement.

The coming out of Jack Andraka was announced via text message.

That's right. I came out via text message. LOL.

I fired off the text to Logan. It was simple, direct, and to the point. "I am gay," I wrote.

The most dramatic moment came before tapping the "send" button. Believe me, that was hard.

Logan didn't act surprised at all to receive my text confession. In fact, she acted like she already knew. She was just happy that I had told her the truth.

That went well! Maybe I was onto something. I told her to spread the word. And she did.

As soon as that text was delivered, I felt a small bit of relief and a lot of terror.

What will my friends say?

What will my teachers say?

Clinging to the chance that this actually might work, I waited. I didn't have to wait for very long. The next day I went to school and the *entire* student body was talking about my sexuality. Instead of winning over my classmates and teachers as I had hoped, it only made me more of a target.

Now it wasn't just students who ignored me, but after word of my sexuality had circulated throughout the faculty room, some of the teachers wouldn't talk to me either. And those times when some classmates did acknowledge my existence, it was to address me by my new name.

Fag.

People called me a fag. Usually behind my back. Sometimes to my face. Looking back, it was hard to tell which was worse. But almost as bad as the name-calling were the persistent looks of disgust I saw out of the corner of my eye every time I walked down the halls.

The jocks were the worst. I avoided them whenever possible, but every week when it came time for gym class, I knew I was in for another round.

"Jack, why are you so gay?" one classmate asked.

"Why are you so bad at math?" I lamely responded.

I'd try to look away and signal that the conversation was over, but it never worked.

"Did you hear about that gay kid that got beat up?" he asked with a glimmer of amusement in his eyes.

I ignored him. But I knew what he was talking about. In school we had discussed a story about a young man who had been beaten up for being gay. He was beaten so severely that he ended up in the hospital. They never caught the people who did it.

"You're next!" he shouted.

There's just no place for me in this world.

I needed to visit Uncle Ted in the worst way. He had been

hospitalized since the beginning of the year. I tried to see him as much as possible, but somehow a few weeks had slipped by without a visit. I hadn't told him of the problems I was having, but now I was thinking it was time to come clean. If anyone could point me in the right direction, it was Uncle Ted. He always knew what to say.

As soon as I walked into the hospital room, I was taken off guard by how dramatically his appearance had changed. Although it had been only four or five weeks since I had last seen him, it looked like he had aged twenty years. All his hair was gone, and he was thin and pale.

"Hi, Uncle Ted."

"Hey, Jack."

He asked about my science projects, and I told him my idea of using bacteria to detect water pollution. I knew he would like that. I didn't mention my troubles in school like I had planned. I just couldn't do it. With the state he was in, I didn't want him to worry about anything else. At the end of my visit, I gave him a hug. He felt like a skeleton. I could feel his shoulder blades poking through his back.

"Jack," he whispered in my ear, "I'm so proud of you."

"I'll see you next week," I told him.

That hospital room experience didn't square with my usual vision of Uncle Ted. Uncle Ted wasn't that sick. I discarded all the evidence and chalked it up to a bad day.

* * *

After coming out as gay and revealing something so personal, I felt totally exposed to the world. There was nowhere to hide. No more masks to wear. Now everyone knew—everyone except my family, that is. A few days after delivering the now-infamous text message, I came home from school to discover my mom waiting at the front door. In my house, the sight of Mom waiting by the door is never a good sign.

"Jack," she said, "do you want to go on a long walk?" That was my mother's way of telling me that she needed to talk to me about something important. We both knew the asking part was nothing more than a formality. It wasn't really a question. It was a command.

I nodded, put my backpack down, and followed her down one of the wooded paths outside our house. My mom got right to the point—one of my classmates heard I was gay and told her parents. The parents called my mom to ask if the rumor was true.

Now my mom wanted to hear it from me. "Jack, is it true? Are you gay?" My mom could always tell when I was lying. I felt frozen. I just couldn't find the strength to meet her eyes. The only safe place to look was down.

What will she think if she finds out the truth?

I willed one foot in front of the other.

Yes, Mom! It's true! I'm gay!!

But the words wouldn't come out.

"Jack, I am ready to walk all night. I want you to answer me," she said.

I knew she wasn't bluffing. My mom didn't bluff. She was stubborn to the core.

I felt defeated. Rock bottom. I had become a joke to my classmates. I didn't really have any friends. I felt as though I did not have much left to lose.

So I told her.

"Yes," I whispered.

"Oh," she said, without a hint of shock or disappointment. "Is that what has been bothering you?"

I was looking at the ground. Leaves and rocks. Rocks and leaves.

"Jack, we don't care about that," she said. "It's part of who you are. I love you."

And that was that. It was no big deal. I was my mother's son. All she cared about was that I was happy.

After hearing it, I realized that I wasn't surprised by Mom's reaction. I had spent so much time telling myself that it didn't matter what my mom thought that I had somehow convinced myself I didn't care whether my mom accepted that I was gay. I was so wrong. Her acceptance mattered to me. Part of me wished I had told her earlier. Maybe she could have helped.

However, I wasn't finished. I still needed to tell my dad. After returning home, I retreated directly to my room. I didn't want to be downstairs when my dad came home. I didn't want to see anyone.

I felt my heart jump into my throat a few hours later when I heard the sound of my dad's car pull up the driveway. It was the sound of inevitability. First the car door opening, then the house door closing. I counted down from fourteen, the number of steps leading up to my bedroom, as he ascended the stairs.

I grabbed a book and pretended I was reading.

He knocked on the door.

"Come in," I said, as if it were just another day.

Of course my mom had told him all about what happened. At least I didn't have to be subjected to that conversation.

He sat down on my bed and asked me to put the book down.

"Jack, I want you to look at me," he said. "I love you, Jack. Just know that you'll always be my son, and I'll always love you."

Like Mom, my dad wasn't upset that I was gay. He also just wanted me to be happy. And I could tell he meant it.

"I know," I said.

I had never asked for his support, but having it meant the world.

Luke, however, was a different story. We barely spoke the first few days after I told my parents, even though I was sure that he knew what had happened. I knew he was busy, so it didn't worry me at first. But once we did start talking, I could tell that something was different. I noticed his sense of humor toward me had changed. He had always picked on me for just about everything, which I knew was to be expected from a big brother, but now there seemed to be a bit of an edge to his jabs.

It was clear to me that Luke was not cool with having a gay brother. Not even a little. This hurt on so many levels. My classmates and teachers were one thing, but I'd always looked up to Luke. His approval meant far more than I'd ever be comfortable letting him know.

One day after Luke had made a particularly hurtful comment, I ran up to my room because I couldn't let him see me cry. I felt miserable and lost.

My mom tried to make me feel better, but she didn't always succeed. One day as we sat in the waiting room at the dentist's office, she told me that I was going to have to toughen up.

"You are going to have to be ready in the event that some people might treat you differently now," she told me.

"What do you mean?" I asked.

"Well," she said, "some parents might have an issue with letting their kids have sleepovers with you and things like that, but don't worry, whatever comes up, we will get through it."

Since Jake and Sam had moved, I didn't have any friends to have sleepovers with, but still, I hadn't even thought about future friends. I began thinking of all the things that could change in my life now that everyone knew I was gay.

During my final stretch of middle school, I thought that I was going to have to live a life completely without real friends. I didn't want to show how much pain I was feeling, so I kicked my cheerful

"I'm gay and amazing" act into full gear.

I buried myself in the world of science and math, which was always an escape for me. After I stopped pretending that I was heterosexual, I also gave up the act that I wasn't into math—as if anyone had believed that anyway! When I was doing an experiment, I didn't have to hide who I was or worry about how others viewed me. It was a safe space where the only things that mattered were my ideas and how well I could execute them.

But no amount of first-place awards could give me relief from the crushing pain I felt every day. After coming out, there was a clique of girls who were nicer to me, but the guys were a different story. They were hell-bent on making sure I never experienced a single moment of peace. And they succeeded.

How's it going, fag?

Are you going to run to the bathroom and cry, Jack?

You know what happens to homos, right?

I tried to remind myself that eventually middle school would end. I was counting down the days.

One afternoon, when my middle school graduation was finally in sight, I came home to find Mom waiting by the door again.

"Jack, sit down," she said. There were tears in her eyes. "There is something I need to tell you."

It was Uncle Ted. He had passed away.

I felt too numb to cry.

It shouldn't have come as a shock, but it did. Uncle Ted had been fighting pancreatic cancer for the past six months and had become very, very sick. But despite all the evidence, I just believed what I wanted to believe: Uncle Ted would find some way to pull through.

I felt my stomach crash down to my feet. In those moments that followed, I felt as though I was looking in on my life from afar. Then the questions came in rapid-fire succession, one after another, but unlike the equations I was used to solving, all the answers seemed so distant, so far out of reach.

Why Uncle Ted? And why did it all have to happen so quickly?

Although I knew how much he had been suffering, in most ways he was the same Uncle Ted, always upbeat and giving great advice. I didn't even get a chance to say a real good-bye. There were so many things I wanted to say—but now it was too late.

How could this have happened?

Only now was I hearing the full story. The diagnosis had come too late. Way too late. By the time he received the news that he was sick, the cancer had already spread. That meant it was too late for surgery to remove the tumors. At that point, everyone knew it would be only a matter of time. Everyone but me, that is.

"Maybe if we had found it earlier." That's what the doctors all said. Now the cancer had taken him. He was gone.

I sat down on my bed and tried to make sense of it all.

Why did this happen?

What am I going to do now?

Why do all these awful things keep happening to me?

It felt like there was nothing firm in my life to hold on to anymore, nothing stable to help me regain my balance. Everything was shifting too fast.

Worse than thinking about all the happy memories I had of Uncle Ted was the thought of all the future moments that the cancer had robbed from me. Now our last moments together, at least in this life, would be spent at his funeral.

When the day came for his service, I was emotionally empty. I didn't cry. I sat there, in a fog, as friends and family took turns saying great things about how bravely he had fought and telling funny stories about him. I was no longer in control of my own body. It was like I was watching from afar as a tiny Jack Andraka walked the line of pews to the casket. On the hour-long car ride home, I couldn't remember a single thing anyone had said. I blankly stared out the window, wondering when I was going to finally wake up from this never-ending nightmare.

I began feeling again the minute I stepped back into my school. A few days after Uncle Ted passed, I was sitting in class when my teacher instructed us to read about this church where the congregants travel around to different parts of the country and stand outside to protest at the funerals of gay people. They hold up these hateful signs spewing venom that the dead gay person is in hell and basically try to do whatever they can to disturb those who are mourning the loss of their loved one.

I kept staring at the words on the page, reading them and rereading them. It didn't make sense.

How could someone . . .

Why would . . .

What the . . .

If you've never felt depression, it's hard to explain. It was as if a massive blanket of hopelessness had draped over me. It was heavy, and no matter how hard I tried, I couldn't shake it off. In a way, I was so depressed that I didn't even want to shake it off and be happy again.

The problem was not just the issues I had faced—the problem was me. I was a hopeless human being, and I couldn't imagine ever arriving at a place where things were better. I wasn't even sure I knew who I was anymore.

The loss of Uncle Ted. The haters. The rejection. Having to hide my sexuality for so long, even the process of coming out, it was all too much for me to handle. I felt like I had exhausted every option. That was it. I was done.

I asked for a pass to the bathroom, walked out of class, and locked the door to the stall. I wanted to hurt myself. I didn't have a knife or anything sharp around me, so I broke off a piece of my pencil and began jabbing the sharp end into my wrists. Again and again. I challenged myself to go farther and farther. To cut deeper and deeper. I wanted to feel more pain. I wanted to see more blood.

I was daring myself to end it. I always was a dare guy. And now I was daring myself to end it all.

The thought of death didn't scare me. Death felt like a relief. If I cut enough, it would all go away. That's really all I wanted.

Everything was becoming a blur. I was in a weird state between numbness and autopilot.

Eventually, I realized I wasn't going to be able to kill myself. The broken pencil wasn't sharp enough. I walked out of the bathroom. Logan and another friend in the hallway saw the bloody marks on my wrists and went straight to the guidance office. A moment later, I was surrounded by counselors.

Next thing I remember, my parents were there at school. After that, it all goes dark.

Chapter 4

THE KNOWLEDGE CURE

After my botched suicide attempt, the school informed my parents that I wouldn't be admitted back until I got some professional help. My parents were equal parts confused and horrified. They were determined to do everything in their power to help pull me out of this abyss.

They found a local LGBTQ (lesbian, gay, bisexual, transgender, and queer) meeting place. They thought it would help if I could talk to other teens who had shared similar experiences, but when I arrived, I was the only teen there. What happened next was a lot of me talking to some random old dude who didn't know me or anything about my deeply personal problems. It's hard to have any kind of healing when you feel awkward and uncomfortable.

Truthfully, I was just sick of talking about it. I wasn't even sure what to say anymore.

What would Uncle Ted say?

He had fought so hard for those extra moments that I was ready to just throw away. If he were sitting next to me today, I thought, he'd begin by asking me about my next project.

More than anything, I really wanted to get back to what I loved—science. There was another science fair coming up, and I had been working on a new idea.

Drawing on my seventh-grade project, I had started on a new one that investigated the effects of metal oxide on certain forms of marine life. This is important because metal oxide is highly toxic and is found in everyday household items like suntan lotion, which often ends up being flushed down our shower drains and into our water supply. I specifically studied its effects on a kind of freshwater plankton called Daphnia magna and the marine bacteria Vibrio fischeri. My results showed that metal oxide behaves differently in marine and freshwater environments. The more we understand about how it interacts with the surrounding environment, the easier it will be to prevent more damage.

But would I even be able to compete? Would I just walk around the rest of my life a damaged head case always in need of attention? As had become the case with seemingly every question, I just didn't know. One thing I did know was that if I wasn't able to rid myself of this heavy blanket of depression, that would mean no more science fairs, no more creek hopping, no more navigating rapids. Nothing.

It wasn't just science that I wanted to get back to. It felt like forever since I'd been on a kayak or white-water rafting. There were so
many rivers I still wanted to explore. I had always wanted to kayak
the Grand Canyon. Would I ever be able to do that?

Then, out of the blue, my brother began to come around. Luke's
favorite lacrosse coach had overheard him making some snide
remark about my sexuality and pulled him aside to tell him a personal story about his own experience in college when he learned that
his roommate was gay. At first he had a lot of the same thoughts that
were probably going through my brother's head—What would people think about him if someone so close to him was gay? How should
he act? But the more time the coach spent with his roommate, the
more he began to see how, no matter what he may have thought of
his sexuality, first and foremost, his roommate was a human being.
And a really cool one at that. The coach told my brother that the two
became lifelong friends.

After the heart-to-heart with his coach, my brother slowly began
to accept me again. He went back to harassing me like he did before
he found out I was gay. Oddly, that went a long way to making me
feel normal again.

Fortunately, I was allowed to enter the science fair. Thank good-
ness, or I wouldn't have graduated and would have been forced to
repeat eighth grade. That was something I wanted to avoid at all

costs. My project, called "A Comparative Study of the Toxicity of Metal Oxides on Vibrio fischeri and Daphnia magna," won first place. It was the third year in a row that I'd finished first overall. It was a huge accomplishment, and I should have been beaming. On the outside, I managed to turn on the smiles. At this point, I had become an expert at faking the emotions people expected me to feel.

I muscled through the last few days of eighth grade and couldn't have been more relieved to walk out of school on the last day. I had no plans to go back.

The start of summer vacation meant math camp. I didn't know what to expect this time. I still had a bad taste lingering in my mouth from my coming-out-to-Anthony debacle after seventh grade. Still, I hoped for the best. Over the past two years, I had seen my two best friends move away, been shunned and humiliated by my classmates, come out of the closet, attempted suicide, and lost one of the people I felt closest to in the whole world. I figured eventually things had to get better because I didn't see how they could get much worse.

This year's camp was being held in Colorado again, where I had had such a great experience after sixth grade. I took this as a good sign. On the first day of camp I met a counselor named Jim. He was smart and I liked the light, easy way that he spoke. Jim didn't seem to have a care in the world. The first weekend of camp, we went on a field trip, and on the bus ride home, I overheard someone mention that Jim was gay. I couldn't believe it. Unlike me, Jim seemed so well adjusted and devoid of any internal chaos. How did he do it? I wanted to learn more. As soon as I got back to my room, I wrote a two-page letter spilling my heart out. I told him about my struggles. About hiding my sexuality. About Anthony. About that day in the bathroom with the pencil. When I was sure no one was looking, I quietly walked to his cabin and slipped the letter under his door.

A few days later, he pulled me aside.

"I got your letter," he said, looking concerned. "Let's talk."

Jim told me his story. He had fought many of the same battles that I had, and he shared his experiences in coming out to his friends and family and overcoming the hatred people felt toward him. Jim was the first person who understood, intimately and personally, what I had been through. But more important than sharing the story of his past, Jim shared with me his hopes for the future. When I looked at Jim, I thought to myself that I, too, could have that kind of future, and more important, that I deserved it.

"Listen, Jack," he said. "You are a smart kid. In the end, it is all going to work out." Jim was the kind of guy who could explain complex math problems in simple language and remain calm in a sea of crazy teenagers. When he said that things would work out for me, I believed him. The two of us talked late into the night.

The last weeks of camp went by too quickly. On our final day, a group of campers and I decided we needed one last adventure. We piled into a car and drove up to Pikes Peak. I didn't have the stomach to look down as the car climbed higher and higher. It was so high that even in the dead of summer, the road was coated with ice and snow. Once we arrived at the top of the 14,115-foot mountain, we jumped out of the car and took positions behind the rocks and trees and started a massive snowball fight. When we were fully drenched with slush and hoarse from screaming and laughing, we retreated to a nearby doughnut shop. We sat, dripping, in one of the booths to dry off while we drank hot chocolate and ate doughnuts. Sitting with my friends, I could see down to the surrounding peaks out the window. For the first time in a while, life felt easy.

That night was filled with long good-byes to all the new friends I had made. Before leaving for the airport, Jim approached me. He had one more piece of advice.

"You have heard a lot about my story and how I got through it," he said. "But Jack, now this is your story. We all have our own paths, but the only one who can decide where it goes from here is you."

Talking to Jim had helped me fully understand that there wasn't anything about me as a person that needed to change. I was done with pretending to be something I wasn't to make other people like me. In accepting that there really was nothing wrong with me, I could deal with the haters in a whole new light. I could choose to ignore them.

I flashed back to the day when I scanned the internet for a

solution. Ignoring the haters was part of the advice I had read, but I hadn't been able to implement it. With the state of mind I was in then, Alan Turing himself, the father of theoretical computer science (and one of my favorite scientists), could have risen from the dead to give me advice and I'm not sure I would have known how to take it.

See, ignoring the haters was the easy part of the solution. The hard part was first refusing to allow my self-perception to be defined by others. Refusing, in other words, to believe that I deserved to be treated differently because I am gay.

Sometimes I still struggle. There are awkward moments, especially at family get-togethers. Some of my extended family have religious views that make them intolerant of my sexuality. To be honest, it's not something we talk about. It's one of those things—I know where they stand and they know who I am. Because we have respect and genuine affection for each other, we leave it at that. For now, that's fine for me.

After landing back in Maryland, I knew there was something else I needed to confront—the loss of Uncle Ted. I hadn't fully realized it, but that initial numbness I had felt since his passing had been replaced by a heavy pain that sat inside my stomach. Now it felt like a big, immovable boulder.

More than anything, I *wanted* to understand why he had died. I *needed* to understand why he had been taken away from me.

And that's when I had an idea. Maybe, just maybe, I could find a cure for pancreatic cancer.

If I had been just a little older and had had time to become a bit more realistic, I probably would have laughed off the idea. After all, I'd hardly be the first person to try, and most of those people were fancy scientists with impressive PhDs from expensive colleges who, unlike me, were old enough to go to an R-rated movie.

There was an older, more mature part of me that knew at the time how ridiculous this all sounded, but the younger, brash part of me was quick to shut him down. Whether it was youthful exuberance or even unbridled stupidity, I didn't know for sure, but whatever the reason, I was all in. Turns out I was the only one.

The first words out of my dad's mouth after hearing my dream were: "Jack, isn't that a little far-fetched?" My parents knew that when I invested myself in an idea, I wasn't a toe-dipper, I was a cannonballer. This probably explains why both of my parents were so dead set against the idea of me dedicating so much of my time to such an impossible task. Especially one that offered such a small chance of reward. After everything I had been through, they weren't exactly sold on the idea of their son leaping into something as heavy as cancer research.

I couldn't really blame them for that one.

However, not having my parents on board was not an option. Their approval was crucial. It wasn't as much about my own morale as it was practical things, like having them drive me places to get supplies or using their credit card to buy stuff online.

Personally, I thought this project was the perfect fit for me—I was in search of an outlet for all my grief, and cancer was in need of a cure. Using everything I learned from giving persuasive speeches to science fair audiences, and also my extreme stubbornness, I began wearing my parents down. Maybe it was the passion I had, or maybe they knew I was going to go ahead and try whether I had their blessing or not, but whatever the case, my parents reluctantly gave me their approval.

Now it was time to begin. I knew from all my time spent working on science fair projects that any discovery begins with identifying goals and then figuring out which questions needed to be answered to get from point A to point B. That part was easy. I already knew what my goal was—to cure pancreatic cancer.

As someone trying to fight cancer of the pancreas, the first question for me was pretty obvious: What the heck is a pancreas? In the beginning, I didn't even know what a pancreas was. I mean, I'd heard of a pancreas and I knew that it was an organ in my body and that it was important, but what exactly does a pancreas do? I had absolutely no idea. I didn't feel intimidated by my lack of knowledge, since I knew I had all the tools I needed to start: Google and Wikipedia.

I started by typing keywords into my laptop—"what is pancreas"—and clicked on the first result that popped up. It was an article on a popular website devoted to health issues, appropriately titled "What Is a Pancreas?"

Turns out the pancreas is actually pretty cool and has *a lot* of responsibilities. The pancreas is a six- to ten-inch-long, spongy, fish-shaped organ located behind the stomach in the back of the abdomen and it produces important enzymes and hormones that help break down foods. Without it, we can't convert the food we eat into the nutrients that we need to survive.

The pancreas also has another huge job. It produces the hormone insulin and secretes it into the bloodstream in order to regulate the body's glucose, or sugar, level. I also learned it has two different kinds of glands. The exocrine glands help speed up chemical reactions and break down fats and proteins. There are also the endocrine glands, which make hormones like insulin that help balance the amount of sugar in the blood. If they aren't working, we get diabetes.

All this information was a lot to digest (get it?). But now that I knew what a pancreas was, I was ready to move on to my next question: What is pancreatic cancer?

After a quick search online, the first thing I realized was that Uncle Ted wasn't the only great person who had fallen victim to pancreatic cancer. This is a particularly lethal form of cancer that has killed a lot of great people, including Steve Jobs, the founder of

Apple. It also took the lives of actor Patrick Swayze, actress Joan Crawford, anthropologist Margaret Mead, and famous opera singer Luciano Pavarotti.

A little farther down, I discovered a story that revealed a disturbing trend: while many different kinds of cancer were becoming less frequent over the past decade, rates of pancreatic cancer have been *increasing* since around the year 2000. The American Cancer Society estimated that 46,420 new cases of pancreatic cancer will be diagnosed in the United States in 2014 and 39,590 people will die that year from the disease.

The lifetime risk of having pancreatic cancer is about one in seventy-eight. It is about the same for both men and women. People get pancreatic cancer when cells in the pancreas begin going wild, growing out of control. Rather than developing into healthy, normal tissue, they continue dividing and form masses of tissue called tumors.

Now that I knew what pancreatic cancer was, I needed to know what caused it. I found a link to a website for Johns Hopkins Hospital. I figured the site had to be credible since it was put together by one of the best hospitals in the world (remember, the information we get from the internet is only as good as its source). I clicked on it.

According to the Johns Hopkins site, doctors and scientists believed there were two main causes of pancreatic cancer. One of those theories was that the damage, or mutations, to our DNA that causes wild clumping in pancreatic cancer might be something we inherit from our parents that is triggered when we get older. But no one seems to know yet whether pancreatic cancer is an inherited disease.

As I researched further, I learned that we have two copies of each gene in our body—one from each of our parents. Scientists believe that people who inherit cancer usually have one mutant copy from one parent and one normal copy from the other parent. As they age, some of these people will damage the good copy of the gene in a cell in their pancreas. That cell will have two bad copies of the gene, and, as a result, that cell in the pancreas will grow into a cancer. These cells just sit like a ticking time bomb until they reach a certain age, when a trigger goes off and the cells begin to mutate.

Pancreatic cancer is considered one of the deadliest cancers in the world. According to the American Cancer Society, for all stages of pancreatic cancer combined, the one-year survival rate is just one in five, and the five-year rate is only 6 percent! That means that only six out of every one hundred people who are diagnosed with pancreatic cancer survive the next five years. You don't have to be good at math to realize that no one in their right mind would want odds like that.

However, reading about those horrible odds led me to another question. How could it be that despite all the new advances in science and exciting breakthroughs in technology, survival rates for pancreatic cancer have remained so astoundingly low?

This is largely a matter of timing. Over 85 percent of all pancreatic cancers are diagnosed late, when someone has less than a
2 percent chance of survival. At this point, the tumors have usually
spread and it is no longer possible to operate and cut them out. Why
is pancreatic cancer being detected so late? Partially, this is because
pancreatic tumors are hard to detect. The pancreas is nestled deep
in the abdomen, beneath other, fragile organs. It also doesn't help
that the pancreas is surrounded by dense, drug-blocking tissue.
Another issue is the test itself. It hadn't been updated in six decades!
The current test is also way too complicated. To screen the blood
of a patient at risk for pancreatic cancer, a doctor must send vials to
a lab, where it can then be tested for elevated levels of a biomarker,
which is a term for an early indicator of disease.

There were more problems. These tests are extremely expensive,
costing eight hundred dollars each. They're also really inaccurate—
missing 30 percent of all pancreatic cancers. While missing only
30 percent is great if you are a major league baseball hitter (that
would mean you are batting .700), it's not so great if you are hoping
to defeat a deadly cancer and a matter of days can mean the difference between life and death.

This meant that one of the biggest problems with pancreatic
cancer wasn't the treatment, but the detection. That's when it hit me.
I didn't need to find a cure for pancreatic cancer. I needed to find a

better way to find pancreatic cancer before it spread to other parts of the body and while it could still be treated. I thought of something the doctors had said after Uncle Ted passed: *Maybe if we had caught it earlier.*

I decided that I had a new mission. I would find an early-detection method for pancreatic cancer.

Unfortunately, there was something else I had to do first—begin high school. On my first day as a freshman at North County High School, I was excited at the prospect of forging a new reputation with a new group of kids, but I was also nervous about having a repeat performance of my middle school years.

The first day began with me slinking from class to class with my head down. Almost everyone had gone to school with one another for the past eight years and already had friends, so no one had any reason to talk to me. All morning I had an ominous feeling that my make-or-break moment would come at lunch. I knew that where I sat would have far-reaching implications for the rest of my future at this school. If I chose wisely, sitting at the right table could help me make important friendships for the rest of the year, or even longer. I was also aware of the dangers. The mistake of unknowingly setting my tray down with the wrong group of students could create the kind of negative first impression that would be hard to overcome.

When the fourth-period bell rang, I walked into the cavernous lunch hall. I was struck by the sheer size of the room. It was so much bigger than the lunch room in my old school. I had become that cliché kid in the movie—the one nervously clenching his lunch tray in his hands as he looks around the room of students, trying to find a safe place to sit down and eat.

I scanned all the different cliques in a desperate search for a safe haven. To the left were the jocks. I remembered them from middle school. No way. To the right were a group of teens wearing designer clothing. They looked okay, but way too hip for me. And besides, there were no open seats next to them. I knew this wasn't good. In standing still, staring, looking like a total weirdo for way too long, I was also putting myself at risk. It was important that I move and move quickly.

I spotted a group of girls sitting near the back of the cafeteria. They were flipping through their books and seemed cool. By their relaxed sense of style and easy smiles, I could tell I would like them. And there was an open seat at their table. I walked over, careful not to dump my tray, and came out with my intro.

"Hi, can I sit here?" I asked.

"Sure," a girl with a nice, welcoming face answered. "I'm Chloe."

Chloe. My savior.

For the rest of the lunch period, I sat in silence, eating quietly. If I didn't say anything at all, I figured, I couldn't say anything wrong. Besides, I was savoring the moment. After all, the ambiance of a high school cafeteria was a step up from my former lunch table, the handicapped stall in the boys' bathroom.

The most important part of the day behind me, I spent the next two hours going through the motions until the final bell rang.

When I wasn't in school, I was hard at work on my project. Now that I had discovered a new goal—finding an early-detection method for pancreatic cancer—I began setting up scientific criteria, a set of rules to work with. In my case, I needed to come up with some ideas as to what the ideal test would have to look like in order to effectively diagnose pancreatic cancer.

I decided that in order to have the kind of impact that could really make a difference, the test would have to be cheap, fast, and simple. My test needed to be sensitive enough to catch the cancer early, but also minimally invasive so it wouldn't bother patients too much. To accomplish this, I knew I'd need a solid plan of action. In science, the defining characteristic of all knowledge, including theories, is the ability to make falsifiable or testable predictions—in other words, predictions that you can prove are either true or false. The specificity of your predictions determines how useful your theory is.

I needed to find some clues that pancreatic cancer leaves in the body to make its presence known. After a lot of searching, I was able to find this great article in a publicly accessible scientific journal called the *Public Library of Science* that listed a database of different proteins that are found in patients suffering from pancreatic cancer.

Why are proteins so important? That wasn't an answer I needed to research online to find. I had learned all about proteins during biology class, in between my torture sessions in middle school. Proteins do most of the work in cells and are required for the structure, function, and regulation of the body's tissues and organs. They are everywhere. 20 percent of the human body is made up of proteins, and they play a crucial role in almost all biological processes.

I also learned that proteins are large, complex molecules made up of hundreds or thousands of smaller units called amino acids, which are attached to one another in long chains. There are twenty different types of amino acids that can be combined to make a protein, and the order of the amino acids determines each protein's unique three-dimensional structure as well as its specific function.

All these proteins in our bodies have very particular reasons and purposes, with each one telling a unique story. Proteins are also good predictors of disease and show up at the earliest stages of every cancer long before the patient feels any symptoms.

One little protein could be the key to detecting pancreatic cancer early, before it spread to other parts of the body and while it was still treatable. I needed to find one that appeared in the earliest stages of pancreatic cancer.

I began to scour the database of proteins. Here, I hit a wall. This wasn't a list of fifteen or twenty proteins that I would have to test.

It was a list of eight thousand! Any one of those unique proteins could be the one! Each one would have to be specifically studied and tested.

That could take a hundred years, and I had already wasted fourteen of them! I turned back to my computer and continued my research. As I worked, I could feel the adrenaline coursing through my veins. If I kept at it, I knew that somewhere within those eight thousand proteins was the answer I was searching for—a biomarker that could potentially save countless lives. Maybe it could even have saved the life of my uncle.

I had no idea if I would succeed.

But one thing was certain: my work had just begun.

Chapter 5
REMEMBER THE PATIENT

It felt so strange to see September come and go without crabbing with Uncle Ted.

Every now and then, I found myself lost in thought, half expecting to look out my window and see his fixer-upper blue sedan swoop down my driveway. I imagined myself sprinting down the stairs, slamming the door behind me, jumping into his passenger seat, and speeding off to begin the dirty work of baiting our crab traps. Few things in life are more disgusting than chicken necks.

Other times, I caught myself replaying the first time I visited him in the hospital after he was diagnosed with pancreatic cancer. I could tell he didn't want to talk about his sickness or the future. I think he knew where that was going. Instead, it was my future that seemed to spark his interest the most. Especially the projects I was working on. Once, when I told him about an idea I had for finding more efficient ways to clean up water, he told me that when times look tough or obstacles appear insurmountable, I should stay focused on who would be affected by my work and all the good it could do.

"In your work, whatever it is you choose to do, never forget who is being impacted," he told me. "Remember the patient."

The advice had hardened into my mind as a sort of living thought memorial.

Remember the patient.

Those words really resonated with me, and not just because it was my uncle's medical condition that first inspired me to wage this battle, but also because those three words served as a stark reminder that our goals extend far beyond ourselves.

In the months that followed the passing of Uncle Ted, my work was fueled by sheer determination. I would come up with an early-detection method for pancreatic cancer, and *nothing* was going to stop me.

It was tedious, and at the end of the day, I had no idea whether any of my hours of hard work were ever going to pay off. I had to sift through thousands of proteins looking for these tiny little differences and asking several questions each time. First, I had to find out if the proteins were down-regulated—meaning that the cell gets smaller in response to an outside change—or up-regulated, meaning that it gets bigger. I needed a protein that was up-regulated, so it would be easier to detect. Once I had finished answering those questions, I had to find out if the proteins were sensitive to all other diseases or only to pancreatic cancer.

Depending on the research I was able to find online, sometimes I was able to rule out a particular protein in a few minutes. But other times, none or very little research was available (at least that I could find), and the process for ruling out just one of these proteins could take hours or even days!

If I was going to follow through with my idea, it was going to take a lot of time and, most important, patience. Patience is an especially important quality if you happen to find yourself haunted by eight thousand proteins every time you close your eyes. Those proteins laughed, did strange dances, and taunted me.

Above all else, it was the false leads that were absolutely killing me. Every few days, I thought I had finally discovered the protein. It seemed to fit all the right criteria, passing every test, and then, just when I got to the point where after spending several hours on it I was about to do the final test to confirm, my hopes would come crashing down.

However, as I was chugging along, working my way through the list of proteins, I noticed that I was beginning to feel seriously worn down. After hours and hours spent staring into screens, it shouldn't have come as much of a surprise.

For a kid who loves the outdoors as much as I do, being trapped in front of my computer all day could sometimes feel like torture. It didn't help that on the few occasions when I had the opportunity to actually see my brother, I had to listen to him drone on and on about all the great things he and his friends were doing without me.

"Then we were just kayaking along and you wouldn't believe what we saw, Jack! A black bear!"

I've never seen a black bear. Lame.

My days at North County High School weren't exactly brimming with inspiration, either. It may have been better than middle school, but I was still a bit shy and I wouldn't have to wait long into the year to learn that my classmates could still be jerks. One day in the beginning of the year, my Spanish teacher went around the room asking the students what they had learned over the summer. Now, here was something I'm comfortable talking about, I thought to myself, as I raised my hand up high.

The teacher called on me and I launched into all the amazing things I had learned over the summer at math camp. In fact, I was too caught up in my own enthusiasm to notice that almost everyone in the class had broken out into a fit of laughter.

I put my head down and felt my stomach sink into my shoes. I felt a flash of heat rise to my face. That was it.

Go ahead and cry, Jack! That will give your classmates four years' worth of ammunition!

Right before the floodgates were about to open, an angry voice of authority cut through the laughter.

"He's new to this school and you think it's a good idea to laugh at him because he likes to learn?" the voice said. "Real mature, guys."

I couldn't believe it! The laughter stopped. I lifted my head and looked around. It wasn't the teacher coming to the rescue. It was Chloe Diggs. The girl who had let me sit next to her at lunch on the first day of school.

It was in that moment that we became friends.

School was easier after that. I sat with Chloe and her friends at lunch and actually talked! She was smart and wanted to hear about the projects I was working on. However, as I became more focused on my task of finding this biomarker, school was becoming less and less relevant to me. I had other matters that needed my attention. I kept reminding myself again and again that I could save one hundred lives a day if I just kept pushing and pushing through protein after protein.

I wish school had been my only obstacle. A lack of money was also testing my already-strained patience. It was shortly after beginning my research that I made the discovery that not all information on the internet is free. Unfortunately for me, that turned out to be especially true for almost all the articles I needed most to move forward with my work.

A lot of the best scientific work available is published in something called a scientific journal. These articles are written by the best of the best in the scientific community. The problem is that the only ones who can access this wealth of information are other scientists—unless, that is, you pay for a subscription. To gain access to one article in a scientific journal will usually cost around thirty-five dollars!

Well, this put me in a tough position. I didn't have any money and my parents could work only so many hours of overtime, but getting the information contained in these subscription journals was absolutely essential for me if I was going to continue my research. I was prepared to try every trick in the book to get my hands on these papers.

First, like any poor teenager, I tried to pirate the papers. But evidently I'm not a very good pirate. And after my feeble career as a hacker crashed and burned, I thought that maybe emailing the professors and doctors who had authored the articles directly and pleading with them to make their work available to me would do the trick. After all, who could resist a kid, right?

It turns out that everyone could resist a kid. Most emailed me back to explain that they didn't own the copyright and weren't allowed to share with the public what they had learned. Others just blew me off entirely.

That's when I resorted to begging my parents for the money. Lucky for me, I am far more skilled at parent-begging than I am at pirating.

If my parents had been less generous, here is where my quest for an early-detection method for pancreatic cancer would have met its end. However, even after my parents agreed to sign off on this high-tech form of highway robbery, my troubles with these articles had only just begun.

Sometimes, I'd go through all that hassle and finally succeed in being able to buy the desired research article, only to discover the pages I had forked over all that cash for had absolutely nothing to do with my research. And as you could probably guess, there was a strict policy of no refunds.

Other times, even when I did manage to get the right article, I found myself staring at the screen for hours like a freak, unable to make sense of all the words. Who wrote these things? More than once the thought even crossed my mind that the scientists writing in these journals were intentionally hoping that no one could read their work.

I began printing out articles. I got into the habit of keeping my computer open and by my side so I could quickly plug words or phrases that I didn't understand into an online dictionary.

Heterozygous.

Hetero means different; *zyg* means yolk or union; *ous* means characterized by or full of. Heterozygous refers to a union character-ized by the joining of two different alleles, or versions of a gene, for a given trait.

It wasn't uncommon for one paragraph to take me half an hour to read. Some days, I felt an overwhelming urge to take all my research, and especially my computer, and make a huge bonfire out in the backyard. I figured we already had enough kindling lying around. Maybe do a new experiment on how quickly accelerants could combust a laptop!

I could visualize myself dancing around the fire and then walking down to my basement/science lab and trashing it in a wild fit of rage. I would take that bat (the one I could never seem to connect with to hit an actual baseball) and just go to town on these awful science projects.

After I had finished on the basement, I would stomp right up the stairs and into my brother's bedroom to demolish all his awards and his science experiments. The thought of it felt . . . so . . . remarkably . . . satisfying.

None of that happened. Instead, I just took a deep breath and pushed on. I kept moving forward, highlighting sections of what I had read that I could understand until eventually more and more words began to make sense to me. Where at first it felt like I was hitting my head against a brick wall, eventually, one by one, a few of those bricks began to fall. After staring at the pages long enough, I was able to actually understand what I was reading in the journals.

Now that I could understand what I was reading, my search for the biomarker moved a whole lot quicker. By the end of October, I

was able to narrow it down from eight thousand to about fifty proteins. That was great, of course, but my work was hardly finished.
While fifty may seem like a manageable number, these weren't
just any proteins. These were the toughest, most time-consuming
proteins of all, in large part because there was almost no research
available on them.

Finally, when I was halfway through my short list and on the
brink of losing my sanity, I came upon a protein called mesothelin. I
ran it through my gauntlet of checklists, cross-referencing it against
all needed criteria in my online database. It was passing test after
test. I held my breath. After so many false hopes, I had been con-
ditioned to keep my enthusiasm at bay until I knew for sure. I kept
pulling up research papers for more information.

Was it up-regulated? Yes!

What body fluid was this protein found in? If it was in spinal
fluid, that wouldn't work. (Ask anyone who has had a spinal tap, and
they will tell you that would not fit my criterion of "easy.") For my test
to work, the biomarker had to be in the blood or urine.

Was it in the blood? Check!

That's it! Mesothelin!

It was the breakthrough I had been waiting for.

I began jumping up and down and screaming for my mother.

"Mom, Mom, it's mesothelin!"

"What?" my mom asked, understandably dumbfounded. "Is

something wrong? Who is mesothelin?"

"No, the biomarker, I found it, it's called mesothelin."

"Oh! I knew you could do it, Jack!" she said. Now she was screaming too. "Does this mean you found the test?"

Well . . . no. But it was a step. A *big* one.

What it did mean was that if someone has pancreatic, ovarian, or even lung cancer, mesothelin is found at very high levels in their bloodstream. But the research papers also indicate that it's found in the earliest stages of the disease, when, if the cancer is detected, someone has close to a 100 percent chance of survival.

As often happens in science, the answer to one problem raised a new question. How did I plan on actually finding this protein in people? I knew that without a way of actually detecting that protein, and, thus, pancreatic cancer, my discovery and all my hard work were essentially useless in the real world.

Again, I scoured the internet and began to print out every article on mesothelin and detection methods that I could find. I became consumed, taking the articles with me to school to read while I was supposed to be working on my class work.

One day shortly after the midway point of my freshman year, I snuck an article on these things called single-walled carbon nanotubes into my biology class. Those are long, thin pipes of carbon that are each an atom thick and one-fifty-thousandth the diameter of your hair. Despite their extremely small size, carbon nanotubes have these amazing properties. They're kind of like the superheroes of material science.

To sneakily read this article during class, I had to be very careful. My biology teacher had this uncanny sense of when I wasn't paying attention. She didn't just have eyes in the back of her head. It was like she had eyes on the sides of her head too.

And while I was reading this article under my desk, we were supposed to be paying attention to these other kind of interesting molecules in the body called antibodies. And these molecules are pretty valuable because they react only with one specific protein and are typically used by your immune system to fight off viruses and bacteria.

And it was then, sitting in class, that it suddenly hit me: I could combine what I was reading about—carbon nanotubes—with what I was supposed to be thinking about—antibodies.

I was having one of those moments when it all began coming together in my mind. I could take these nanotubes and mix them with antibodies (think of it as putting meatballs in some spaghetti) so that you have a network that reacts with only one protein—in this case, mesothelin. When the mesothelin reacts with the antibody, they form a larger molecule called an immunocomplex (imagine a super-beefed-up protein molecule). When this gigantic molecule is formed, it actually separates neighboring nanotubes and causes the network to spread, akin to taking a bundle of wires and pulling it apart. When this happens there are fewer connections between the neighboring nanotubes and so there are fewer pathways for electrons to take when traveling through the network, increasing the electrical resistance! So the electrical properties of the nanotubes would change, and that was something I could measure.

I could feel the simple pleasure of all these puzzle pieces linking together in my head . . . and then . . . Busted! In the middle of my breakthrough, there was my biology teacher storming up to my desk. She had that angry look on her face. Again.

Be cool, Jack.

"Mr. Andraka!" she shouted.

From the moment I first walked into her classroom, it had been obvious that this teacher didn't like me. I asked too many questions. I didn't always do things the same way her textbook instructed.

I frantically began formulating my response, but before I had time to answer, she snatched my paper on carbon nanotubes out of my hand and held it up in the air with disdain as if waving around a porn magazine.

"What is this?" she snarled.

It's a science paper. Shouldn't that be a good thing? I wanted to say, but didn't.

"It's just a science article," I answered.

She responded with another disgusted look and walked away with the contraband science article.

Are you kidding me? Great!

She deposited my science paper in the dark recesses of her desk. I knew what this meant. There was only one way to get my paper back. I would have to wait until after class, approach her desk, and beg.

Time to swallow your pride, Jack.

After the bell rang, I approached. That was when I had to sit and endure her long-winded lecture on "respect." I wasn't respecting her class. I wasn't respecting her lesson. I had no respect for anything. I was very disrespectful!

While she was speaking, I may have been reacting physically, nodding at the appropriate time, but I was in a different world, caught up in the excitement of my idea.

This is it!

Mashing these antibodies into a network of carbon nanotubes should work, at least in theory. However, there was a problem. These networks of carbon nanotubes are extremely flimsy and they needed to be supported. After school, I went straight home, sat on the floor of my room, and began brainstorming.

Hmmm . . . what is something that is cheap but could also offer a little support? I know, paper!

This should be easy. You start with some water, pour in some nanotubes, add antibodies, mix it up, take some paper, dip it, dry it, and you can detect cancer in seconds, long before it becomes life-threatening. And because of the cheap materials needed, it would cost only pennies!

Then, suddenly, a thought occurred to me that thwarted my brilliant plan. There was absolutely no way my mom was going to allow me to do cancer research on my kitchen countertop or even in my basement. I also didn't have the right equipment my task required. I needed to be in a real laboratory.

I consulted the internet. I learned that the only way a fourteen-year-old kid like me could get access to a fancy laboratory is to first create a step-by-step written description of the idea and plan, called a proposal, and send it out to every doctor who specialized in pancreatic cancer and hope one of them believed in my idea enough to accept me.

The next four months of my life were spent working on an experimental design and a proposal for my theory. It was harder than honors biology. My proposal had to be over thirty pages long and include a budget, a materials list, a timeline, pitfalls, and reagents, which are substances used in chemical analyses. I described my theory of lacing mesothelin-specific antibodies in painstaking detail.

Once I had completed the finishing touches on my proposal, I went online to all the directories at local universities and compiled a master list of all the doctors who were in a position to accept me. I figured after I got back their acceptances, I would have to choose which laboratory I thought would be the best fit. That should be fun!

Over the next forty-eight hours I fired off my scientific proposal to two hundred different professors at places like Johns Hopkins University and the National Institutes of Health—essentially anyone who had anything to do with pancreatic cancer. And I sat back waiting for these positive emails to pour in, saying, "You're a genius! You're going to save us all!"

And I waited.

And waited.

And waited.

Chapter 6

FAILING UPWARD

The next day I was standing in front of my locker, about to grab my books for fifth-period biology class, when Damien approached. Unfortunately, Damien was one of a handful of classmates who had moved along with me to my new high school.

"Yo, Jack," he said, patting me on the shoulder. "What have you been working on lately?"

I knew there was only one reason this kid was being nice to me. Given my track record of recent science fair success, I figured he was fishing for information.

I chalked it up to desperation. After all, it was freshman year. That meant, for the first time, the winner of our local science fair would be eligible to qualify for an all-expenses-paid trip to *THE* Intel International Science and Engineering Fair. Or as those who worshipped science called it, ISEF.

Two years had gone by since that incredible and eye-opening trip to San Jose, California, when, as a seventh grader, I had watched Luke walk up onstage to accept his special award. After bearing witness to the most elite teen minds in the Milky Way, it made the totality of my accomplishments feel small in comparison. While my time at ISEF was educational and invigorating, it also left me feeling bereft. It was as if I had been handed the most spectacular bacon cheeseburger and, after taking one tiny bite, had it ripped from my jaws. I still had that ISEF taste in my mouth, and I wanted more.

Damien was standing a few feet to my left, studying my face for clues.

"Oh, nothing much," I told him with a shrug. "Still just trying to come up with something." I'm a terrible liar.

"That sucks," he said. "Because this is the year you're going down, Andraka."

"Yeah, right," I responded.

I knew my comeback was lame, but I didn't care. Trash-talking was never a strength of mine. Besides, I decided I'd let my project speak for itself.

However, if my science project was going to be worth its weight in nanotubes, I was going to need to secure that laboratory—and fast. After the final bell rang, I hurried straight home, hopeful that an email would be waiting for me with the news that I was accepted into a laboratory. I checked my inbox—nothing.

There's no need to worry, I told myself. *Doctors are busy people.*

I hung out a lot in front of my computer that first night. When I wasn't hitting the refresh key every few seconds, I passed the time by studying the pictures that the doctors had posted of themselves on their hospital profile pages. I couldn't help but notice how inviting they all looked.

The next day when I came home from school, I had finally received my first response.

I opened it.

Thank you for inquiring about space at our laboratory for your research; unfortunately . . .

It was a rejection in the form of one of those automated responses. I didn't need to read any more.

"That's strange," I told myself, shrugging it away. "I guess she just didn't get it."

Later that day, my dad and I took a trip to the Chesapeake Bay to do a test run on the carbon paper strips. We wanted to see if the strips were sensitive enough to detect E. coli in the bay. The test worked, and, unfortunately for those who depend on the bay for their water supply, we detected large quantities of the deadly bacteria.

When I got home that night, there was another rejection.

Thank you for inquiring about space at our laboratory for your research; unfortunately . . .

This wasn't making sense. I opened up my proposal and checked it for errors. Everything checked out. Perhaps, I thought, I had made some horrible mistake in my introductory cover letter.

Dear Dr. So and So,

I am a high school student who attends North County High School. I am currently doing a science fair project on the use of nanotubes and antibodies to detect pancreatic cancer (strain RIP1). For my project, I plan on producing my antigens and antibodies through the immunization of mice with MUC1. The MUC1 will be derived from xenografted RIP1 in mice and will be extracted using a hot phenol: water extraction procedure. My procedure is attached to this email. I was wondering if I could work in your laboratory to produce MUC1, which will then be used to produce PAM4. Thank you for your time, your research is absolutely amazing. If you cannot help me can you refer me to someone who can.

Sincerely,

Jack Andraka

I thought it worked. It was straightforward with just the right touch of flattery. However, on this second read, I did notice a problem with the last sentence—I had placed a period where I should have placed a question mark. Ugh.

During the week that followed, a third rejection letter arrived. And a fourth. And a fifth.

Thank you for inquiring about space at our laboratory for your research.

We regret to inform you that we are unable to make space available.

Thank you and best of luck on your research.

Again, my youthful optimism held firm. *Maybe they didn't read it. I mean, it is thirty pages long,* I told myself. I still had a vast majority of doctors evaluating my proposal, all of whom could still give me lab space. But like an airborne virus on a transcontinental airplane, the rejections continued multiplying in my inbox.

I'd like to help, but the lab is really full of students. We just cannot take any more.

Another lesson I learned—the doctors' appearances in their hospital profile pictures don't always match up with their dispositions.

Dear Mr. Andraka,

While your idea initially sounded very exciting, the procedure was a far cry from something bearing any significance in our field. Before you continue wasting any more precious time of my

fellow researchers I suggest you better educate yourself in your
field of interest.

That one hurt.

A small consensus was forming among doctors in the field of pancreatic cancer research that was becoming impossible to ignore: Jack, this is the worst idea *ever.*

After the first fifteen days, I began to dread logging on to my computer and checking my inbox. Being told your idea sucks is bad enough, but even worse was the knowledge that every rejection meant there would be one less opportunity to achieve my goal. I began to keep a running tally. At the three-week point, the score looked insurmountable since 114 people had turned me down. Not one had accepted me.

At lunch the next day, I vented to Chloe about all my rejections. It's a firmly held belief of mine that it is rude to complain while eating, but I just couldn't help myself.

"I don't care," I said. "I don't care about any of it."

I pulled out the peanut butter and jelly sandwich that my mom had packed and took an angry bite.

"It's because I'm younger," I continued. "These doctors can't get past my age. They can't get past the fact that I'm a kid. They don't care about my ideas, they just don't want to babysit me."

I looked up at Chloe. It hadn't taken us long to find out all the things we had in common, most important a curiosity about nature and a stubborn belief that we would make anything out of life that we wanted. Chloe also happened to be a great listener, which at the moment I really appreciated.

"I'm tired of everything and everyone," I continued, my voice getting louder, beginning to tip with rage.

"Jack," she said, her eyes full of compassion as she placed her hand over mine. ". . . You have jelly on your face."

I lost it. We both cracked up. Sure, I was stressed, but in the moment I was also grateful. Middle school was over, and I was spending lunch sitting at an actual table, across from a good friend.

But I still had not had any positive responses to my email. I had given it all I had. I had sent my best proposal to every doctor in a position to give me lab space. It was clear that no one was taking my ideas seriously. There was no Plan B. I hadn't thought that far ahead.

My parents began to worry. They chose a lazy Sunday morning to sit me down for a talk. My dad is so practical that he got right to the heart of the matter: they just didn't think my idea would work, and they were concerned that the disappointment would be too much for me to handle. I was exhausted, trying to look attentive despite having driven myself crazy going over my proposal again and again in search of whatever it was that was turning the doctors off.

My parents had lots of arguments. All I had were three little words.

"But it works."

After a lot of me listening to them talk, my parents gave each other a long look.

"If you feel this strongly," my dad said, "we can keep going."

It was hard to argue with the points that my parents had brought up. Almost two hundred of the most distinguished doctors in the world had seen my proposal, many of whom had studied pancreatic cancer their entire careers, and without exception, they all said no. Despite giving me their blessing to move forward, it was now clear that my parents weren't convinced my idea would work, either. Did anyone actually believe in this project besides me?

I began to question if I even believed in my project. Maybe I had missed something. Maybe if I just went over the proposal one more time. Or a hundred.

As the week went by, six more responses came—all rejections.

Now I felt desperate. I made the risky and somewhat terrifying decision to approach my older brother.

There wasn't a mind in the world I respected more than Luke's. That is why I needed to talk to him. I knew that not only would he be honest with me, but he would probably be right.

However, as I walked over to him I felt like I was headed toward the guillotine. After handing him my proposal and walking him through all my conclusions, I carefully watched over his shoulder as he scanned through the pages. As he read, he occasionally paused, looking up as if deep in thought.

After he had flipped through the last page, I braced myself and waited for him to crush my dreams with the ruthlessly sharp logic of his mind.

Then, I heard a strange grunting noise followed by a pause. I waited.

"This works," he said.

I held my breath, waiting for the zinger that was sure to come next, but instead he just repeated it to himself.

"This works."

"It will work," he added, this time with emphasis.

His words hit me like a shot of adrenaline straight into my heart. I felt the impulse to jump in the air and fist-bump the ceiling, but my pride wouldn't allow it. Instead, I played it cool.

"I know," I said casually as I pulled the copy of my proposal out of his hands and walked into the kitchen to get a snack. "Just double-checking."

From that moment forward, I didn't doubt the validity of my idea again.

In May, one month and 192 rejections later, I came home from school, opened my inbox, and braced myself for the knockout punch that was sure to come.

The subject line read: "A message from Dr. Anirban Maitra."

This is a really interesting proposal. Come in and talk about it.

Not sure I could trust my eyes, I read over the words again.

Come in and talk about it.

"Mom!" I screamed.

My voice must have echoed more with terror than triumph, because my mom and Luke rushed over to see the image on the screen in front of me.

"Jack?" she said.

"Look."

One, two, three . . .

They both erupted in a roar!

"That's awesome," Luke said, patting my shoulder. "You got this."

This wasn't just any doctor. Dr. Anirban Maitra of Johns Hopkins in Baltimore was one of the preeminent scientific minds in the world on the subject of pancreatic cancer. I understood I hadn't been accepted, but it was a foot in the door.

My next step was to learn *everything* about him.

I went online and studied his résumé. It read longer than my former list of proteins: Professor of Pathology and Oncology, the Sol Goldman Pancreatic Cancer Research Center; Affiliate Faculty, Department of Chemical and Biomolecular Engineering; Affiliate Faculty, McKusick-Nathans Institute of Genetic Medicine. Dr. Maitra was the cream of the crop.

His specialty of study was how to best utilize specific biochemical differences between cancer and normal cells so that the effects of chemotherapy harm only the cancer cells, not the healthy ones. He was also working on revolutionary approaches for identification of abnormal pancreatic cancer genes using cutting-edge "gene chip" technologies that would allow scientists to query multiple genetic loci—including, in some instances, the whole human genome—for abnormalities that are unique to pancreatic cancer but not present in normal tissues. I might not have understood exactly what all that meant, but I knew enough to know that I would be in the presence of greatness!

An interview was scheduled for two weeks later. When the big day came, I felt vaguely ill. All those rejections had done a number on my confidence. I knew that my science was sound, but I was nervous about whether I'd be able to express my ideas effectively.

The hospital was located in Baltimore, which is about a thirty-minute drive from my home. It was a quiet car ride. I was replaying all the main talking points I didn't want to forget.

By mashing the antibodies into a network of carbon nanotubes, I will be able to identify a single protein, which in this case is mesothelin, that will serve as a biomarker for pancreatic cancer. By using carbon paper, I will have something strong enough to support the flimsy carbon nanotubes.

I hugged my mom as she dropped me off at the hospital's front door.

"You'll do fine, Jack, just be yourself," she said.

I walked inside the hospital and introduced myself to the receptionist. "Hi, I'm Jack Andraka."

I gave her my biggest smile. She gave me a look: the same one a bank teller wears before offering a lollipop.

"I'm here to see Dr. Maitra," I added.

"Sure, come this way," she said. She led me down a hallway. There would be no lollipop.

I concentrated on my own feet. No tripping. Not here. Not now.

She stopped in front of an office. Through the door, I could see fancy plaques on the walls. Inside, waiting, was Dr. Maitra.

He introduced himself. I shook his hand.

"Hi, Jack, it's so nice to meet you."

The man looked true to his picture. He had a naturally inquisitive and cautious smile.

Dr. Maitra had an aura of wisdom. He spoke slowly and deliberately, and my first impression was that he was patient and sincere.

"I was very impressed by your proposal," he said. "Remarkable for someone of your age."

I felt a renewed confidence as I explained my process and walked him through how I came to each one of my conclusions. As I spoke, he nodded occasionally.

Everything seemed to be going well. But just as I thought we were wrapping up the interview and had braced myself for the words I had been waiting to hear—that he was going to give me some space in his laboratory—he said, "Come this way, please."

I was ushered into a small conference room where, out of nowhere, all these doctors began appearing, as if by spontaneous generation. The gaggle of doctors began firing questions at me left and right!

I dug in. I hadn't come all this way only to stumble a few feet short of the finish line. Some of the answers I knew. Others, I just kind of improvised.

Question: "How did you come to your conclusion that mesothelin was the biomarker?"

Answer: "I went through researching each individual protein, one by one, until finding one that matched the criteria."

Question: "How did you reach your conclusion that nanotubes would be effective?"

Answer: "I realized I could take nanotubes and mix them with antibodies to create a network that only reacts with mesothelin."

They were relentless. It was exhausting. I felt like I had aged a year during the two-hour interrogation.

Finally, it was over. I had survived. I studied the faces of the doctors. They seemed pleased.

Next came the words I had been longing to hear.

"Okay, let's do this," Dr. Maitra said.

I would be able to use his laboratory. Actually, he agreed to let me use a small corner of the laboratory, and he assigned me one of his assistants to make sure I didn't blow the place up—but all things considered, I was in business. It was clear that Dr. Maitra was an exceptional doctor, but the fact that someone with his standing in the medical community was willing to take the ideas of a kid seriously told me he was also an exceptional person.

My mom, who had been waiting all those hours outside the hospital in the Andraka family station wagon, was staring at the front door as I walked outside.

I gave her a thumbs-up and ran over to her.

"I knew you could do it, Jack!" she screamed through the open driver's-side window.

"When do you start?"

"Ten days."

Even though I physically spent the next week at school, mentally I was in my new laboratory, rehearsing my procedure step by step. Since I had already discovered the protein, mesothelin, and found a way to test for it with my paper strips, I was confident that the most difficult part of my journey was now behind me. *This should take a day*, I assured myself. *Two days, max.*

My dad had already helped me build a Plexiglas testing apparatus that I could use to hold the strips as I read the currents. I grabbed a pair of my mom's sewing needles to use as electrodes. I was taking full advantage of my parental resources.

On my first day at the lab, I learned something new. I was absolutely *horrible* at doing research.

It was only a few hours after my mom dropped me off for my first day in the laboratory when I contaminated my experiment by sneezing on my vials of cells.

Seriously. I sneezed on them! Who does that?

I was so ashamed that I hid my mucus-covered tray of contaminated cultures in between a bunch of different flasks so no one would see my amateur move. Destroying something with a sneeze might sound humorous, until you realize that it means hours of hard work wasted all because I forgot to turn my head or bring a tissue. However, that wasn't the only time my sneeze brought me to tears. It wasn't long after that I had another nasal calamity.

I had carefully created my carbon nanotubes, which look like black tomato soup, and placed the little tubes on a bench. Then it happened again. The force of my sneeze knocked them off a bench and smashed them onto the floor.

This time, there were other scientists in the room. Everyone stared at me as I watched the black spot spread across the floor. I felt like such an idiot. One thing about nanotubes that most people don't realize is that they stain. The custodians who came in at night had no idea what to do with my mess. To this day, the stain is still there, a permanent reminder.

I thought I was doing better until, twelve weeks after beginning at the lab, I clumsily tripped over the untied laces of my red sneakers and stumbled into my culture cell test tubes. I watched helplessly as they all crashed into the floor. It had taken me two months to grow the MIA PaCa-2 cells, which would replicate the pancreatic cancer cells in my test. Now I would have to start from scratch.

My mom had always pestered me about my shoelaces. *You let those laces dangle and one day you are going to regret it, Jack.*

Did I ever.

However, all my problems paled in comparison to my struggles with the Western blot. The Western blot, which is also sometimes called the protein immunoblot—or, as far as I was concerned, evil incarnate—is a machine that uses something called gel electrophoresis to separate proteins by their 3D structure or length. The proteins are then transferred to a membrane where they are stained with antibodies specific to the target protein.

If that hurts your head to read, try actually doing it. The precise measurements and care needed for every step were like a game of Operation. Every time I made the smallest mistake, or miscalculated in the slightest way, I had to junk the rest of my work and start over again.

Then, if I ever managed to successfully master the Western blot, I would be confronted with the equally difficult task of mixing the human mesothelin–specific antibodies with single-walled carbon nanotubes, which I used to coat strips of filter paper to make the paper conductive.

The next step involved using a scanning electron microscope to determine the optimal layering of the paper. If I hadn't messed up by that point, the MIA PaCa cells should have spiked with varying amounts of mesothelin and could then be tested against the paper biosensor. I only saw the results of my experiment once I had graphed out the measurements of electricity on the paper test strips. It should reveal exactly how much of the biomarker protein mesothelin was in the blood.

Most days I thought I would never get it right. If I wasn't contaminating my experiments with my sneezes or knocking them over, I was accidentally baking my cultures in an incubator.

Since I was the youngest in the lab, I didn't have much to add when the doctors talked about their spouses and kids, and I was ashamed of my performance. I was embarrassed by the black stain on the floor and the fact that I called the forceps "tweezers," which made them laugh. When the doctors pulled chairs up around a table near the lab, I took my food to a stairwell. It was better than eating in the middle school bathroom.

As I ate in the stairwell, I remembered the 192 doctors who rejected me, and I wondered if Dr. Maitra had begun to regret the day when he gave me space in his lab.

Maybe I am Dr. Maitra's charity case.

Sometimes, after coming home from the lab, I'd find another rejection letter.

Dear Mr. Andraka,

After spending time reviewing your idea, it is clear that you
should consider a few more years of education.

Sincerely,
Dr. So and So

The more I worked, the more I saw that there were countless holes in my original theory. After five grueling months in the laboratory, the only thing I had to show for my efforts was the hockey puck–sized stain of nanotubes on the floor.

One day, I went to my secret spot under the stairwell and broke down in tears. I felt like the unluckiest scientist in the world. That night, I went home and reread a passage online about legendary inventor Thomas Edison.

On December 10, 1914, ten entire buildings full of Edison's treasured experiments were engulfed in flames and destroyed. Much of Edison's life's work turned to ash that night. He was sixty-seven years old, and many believed that Edison's days as a great American inventor had gone up in smoke too.

However, as he stood watching the flames burn away years of records and prototypes, Edison turned to a reporter from the *New York Times* and told him, "Although I am over sixty-seven years old,

I'll start all over again tomorrow. I am pretty well burned out tonight. But tomorrow there will be a mobilization here and the debris will be cleared away, if it is cooled sufficiently. I will go back to work to reconstruct the plant. There is only one thing to do," Edison continued, "and that is to jump right in and rebuild."

Edison even took it a step further, and began to explain how the fire was actually a great opportunity. Now that "the rubbish" of his old factory had been burned away, he could begin the task of building a bigger factory that would be better than the old one, he told his son. With that, he rolled up his coat for a pillow, curled up on a table inside one of the buildings in the burned-out factory, and fell asleep. When Edison woke up he looked at the ruins and said, "There is great value in disaster. All our mistakes are burned up. Thank God we can start anew." With that, he immediately began the task of getting his plant up and running again. His employees worked double shifts and set to work producing more than ever.

It wasn't just Edison's innate genius that separated him from the other scientists of his day. What I love about that passage on Edison is it shows his ability to see missteps as stepping-stones. Three weeks after the fire, Edison invented the phonograph, the first device to record and play sounds.

I began to see that although many of the mistakes I was making were the result of inexperience, other times, like in the case of the Western blot, my errors taught me to be more careful and pay closer attention to the details of my work. I made a conscious effort to see the setbacks as opportunities and to remind myself that within each mistake was a clue that could bring me another step closer to creating an early-detection method for pancreatic cancer.

During these days the words of Uncle Ted were never far from my mind.

Just slow down, Jack, you're going to be okay. Everything will work out.

I dug in my heels and began working longer hours, every day after school and past midnight on Saturdays. I barely ate. When I did remember that I needed food, my diet consisted of pizza, hard-boiled eggs, and Twix candy bars. I worked through Thanksgiving and Christmas. When I needed sleep, I snuck under the stairwell, where I had made a mattress out of magazines and copies of printed-out journal articles, and, using my hoodie as a pillow, took a quick power nap. I thought it was a great hiding space until, one time, I woke up from a nap and saw Dr. Maitra staring down at me with a look of complete confusion.

"Hi, Dr. Maitra," I said.

"Hi, Jack," he answered. He walked away shaking his head.

For my fifteenth birthday, I brought a bunch of party hats and colorful streamers from the dollar store and decorated my workspace with signs congratulating myself. It was a weekend and the laboratory was empty.

One night in late December, after seven long, grueling months in the laboratory, I was having a particularly hard time. No matter how hard I tried, I just couldn't seem to get through the procedure without making a mistake.

I had memorized my procedural checklist (which is kind of like a recipe) and kept a tissue close by in the event of any unexpected sneezes.

The first thing I always had to do was make sure that I had all the right ingredients on hand:

1. Mesothelin protein
2. A dozen test tubes in a carrier
3. Phosphate buffer solution, a water-based salt solution containing sodium phosphate and sodium chloride
4. A pipette, which is a chemical dropper that looks like a big syringe
5. A dozen of my custom-made nanotube-soaked paper sensor strips, each about half the size of a pinky
6. An ohmmeter, a device that measures electric currents

Once I had everything, I was ready to get to work.

First, I needed to combine the carbon nanotubes, which look like a black powdery soot and weigh about one gram, with the antibodies by pouring both into test tubes and mixing them together.

It wasn't easy. Carbon nanotubes stick together and form bundles, which have to be unzipped by hitting them with ultrasound waves called sonication. The ultrasound waves create vibrations that make these bundles tear apart so they can be used for testing.

Next I made my testing strips by taking some pieces of filter paper and cutting them into strips measuring five centimeters by a half centimeter before dipping them into my nanotube-antibody soup. Each strip had to be dipped and dried thirteen times. My first batch took twenty hours to make because the humidity in the air had added extra moisture. Eventually, I learned a way to make them dry

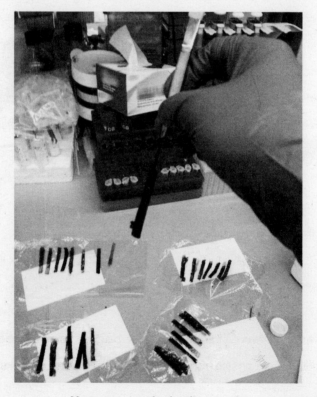

My test strips, coated with carbon nanotubes

more quickly by placing them in a vacuum tube to suck all the water out. It is the same process they use to make astronaut food.

After the test strips were dry, I put my mesothelin sample on the soaked carbon paper to see if the protein would react to the antibody network. To see my results, I put electrodes on my strip and used my ohmmeter to measure the electric pulse. The process was painstaking. Every little step in my test was time-intensive and had to be absolutely flawless. Now, if my theory was right, the readings would show that the antibodies on my paper strips had detected my biomarker.

I furiously worked out the math equation. I made a graph of the measurements of the electrical currents along with the various amounts of individual protein solutions to find something called a dose-dependent response, which would basically see how they all matched up. I only knew if I had made a mistake after completing an entire batch.

I screwed up my first batch and had to start over. Then I contaminated my second batch, too. Three more hours spent creating the third batch resulted in more failure.

All the while, my mom was outside waiting in the parking lot. It was getting late. I was tired. *Maybe I should just call it a night*, I thought.

I decided to give it one more try. For the fourth time, I began the tiresome procedure of making my batch of solutions, sucking up some of the protein from my vials with my pipette, dropping the proteins on my nanotube-soaked paper test strips, and then hooking up my ohmmeter to my paper test strips and running the numbers.

Wait! What is this?

As I began graphing the amounts, something was different. The numbers showed that my test with little papers strips had detected the biomarker!

I ran the numbers again. It was working. The ohmmeter was measuring the mesothelin levels in the solutions!

My test had showed a direct correlation between how much protein was in the solution and how much the electrical properties were changing. That meant its sensitivity was good enough to detect pancreatic cancer. My results were passing all the preliminary tests!

Holy crap! It's working?

Overwhelmed with hysterical joy, I ran around the small lab in circles, screaming like a hyena and trying not to knock anything over. Then a thought occurred to me—*It's so late at night. What if I saw what I wanted to see and not the actual results?*

I ran back over and checked my results again. My hands were shaking as I held the ohmmeter. There it was—my hypothesis was correct.

I did it?

I wanted to share the moment with someone, anyone, but looking around the empty laboratory, I realized that it was 2:30 a.m. on a Sunday, and everyone else had gone home hours before.

My mom! I need to see my mom.

I had forgotten about my poor mother! She was still parked outside, probably asleep in the car, waiting for me. I went into full-sprint mode until reaching her.

"Hey, Mom, guess what?" I said, a wide smile across my face.

Barely awake, my mom opened her eyes and smiled back at me. She groaned.

"It's working!" I screamed at her.

She didn't answer with words. She began screaming. I was screaming. We were both screaming.

My mind raced through all the implications of the achievement. My paper sensor cost less than a nickel and would take five minutes to run, making it faster, cheaper, and more sensitive than the current test. It could save lives, lots of them.

I felt like I was dreaming. Yelling back and forth with my mom at the top of our lungs on the car ride home will go down as one of the best memories of my life. I felt as though I could lift off the ground.

However, as we pulled into the driveway I began to feel a small stab of pain. The one person I wanted to share my joy with more than anyone else was Uncle Ted. I would have picked up the phone and woken him up. He would have loved this moment most of all.

I wanted to stay up all night thinking about the future, about what this discovery would mean, but I needed sleep. After all, I had to go to school the next day.

Chapter 7
CANCER PAPER BOY

When my alarm went off the next morning, I was wearing the same hoodie as the day before. I was not convinced that I had slept at all. And then the events of the day before struck me like a bolt of lightning, zapping me out of bed.

Did it happen?

Did I dream it?

Did I really make a test that works?

I unzipped my backpack, which was sitting beside my bed, pulled out the notebook I used to graph my calculations, and began flipping through the pages.

There it was! My graph of the measurements of the electrical currents.

I pulled out my calculator and ran the numbers again. They all checked out.

I ran downstairs. My dad was standing in the kitchen, giving me a knowing look.

"Late night?" He smiled at me over his newspaper.

It was—and it wouldn't be the last.

Just because I had detected mesothelin in artificial samples didn't mean my work at the lab was finished. I still needed to find out if my test would show my biomarker in human pancreatic tumors, too.

I fired off an email to Dr. Maitra, letting him know about my findings in the artificial samples and, more important, that I needed new supplies to begin testing for human tumors. He agreed to set me up with what I needed, but not before telling me how proud he was of my success.

Wow, great job, Jack, this is really exciting, he wrote.

However, this next step wouldn't be without drama. We had to use live mice. As a ferret owner, I am easily attached to anything small and fury. The worst part of the entire experience may have been when we needed to euthanize the mice with gas. I couldn't be in the same room. I had to walk down the hall.

In January I was able to replicate in the human samples what I had done with the artificial ones. Now it was time to shift gears. This year the International Science and Engineering Fair was going to be held on May 12, in Pittsburgh, Pennsylvania. That meant I had four months to prepare.

I'd been dreaming about that competition for years. As the world's largest high school science research competition, to me it was like the Super Bowl, World Series, NBA Finals, Stanley Cup, and Olympics all rolled into one and multiplied by a factor of three.

But ISEF is *way* more than just some big science fair—it is also a huge six-day celebration of science, math, and technology, where young scientists get together to talk about and share their ideas and experiences. Basically, my concept of heaven on earth.

The competition at ISEF is fiercer than anything I have ever experienced. The field of contestants is pulled from seven million high school students from around the globe. Only the 1,800 winners of local, regional, state, and national competitions are invited to participate. All these kids bring mind-blowing projects deserving of recognition. I couldn't think of a better venue anywhere in the world to showcase my new discovery.

As soon as I had wrapped up my work at the lab, I began the task of preparing my findings for the science fair circuit. A good presentation was one that took complicated science and turned it into a story that engages people. And I didn't want merely a good presentation; I wanted a great one. I titled my project "A Novel Paper Sensor for the Detection of Pancreatic Cancer."

Before I brought my project to ISEF, I wanted more practice. I began to research other science fairs, trying to find ones that fit my schedule so I'd have enough time to prepare and coordinate travel. I tried to hit as many as possible to practice for ISEF.

I went first to the Hopkins Science Competition. I had never been, but knew it had a sterling reputation. The fair was a great test to see how my project measured against stiffer competition. Here I went head-to-head with a lot of brilliant graduate researchers who were much more experienced and older than I was.

After setting up my display, I began to see many familiar faces, but I couldn't place them. All of a sudden I realized that I was recognizing the doctors who had rejected me. There they were, milling around the convention floor and supporting many of my competitors who were under their tutelage. Others were even working as judges.

My face turned red with anger. I flashed back to some of the rude rejection letters that trashed me and my ideas. I wanted them to know that I wasn't just some child who had been wasting their time. My ideas mattered too. At the awards ceremony, I had convinced myself that the deck was stacked against me. I thought the merit of my findings would be overlooked because of my young age. I was shocked when they announced that I had won. Judging by the look on my parents' faces, I wasn't the only one.

Maybe, I thought, these doctors weren't as bad as I thought. I lingered a little longer than I should have, hoping that one would offer congratulations on my victory. Not one did.

It was great to get that victory, but, more than anything, I was focused on ISEF. I knew that if I was to have any hope of pushing my project out of the world of theory and onto pharmacy shelves, where it could actually help people, I needed some help from the mainstream science community.

I was proud of all my middle school projects, but the truth was that not one had actually been implemented in the real world yet. Maybe, I thought, if other scientists could see what I had done with pancreatic cancer, they could help push my project up the ladder.

Meanwhile, at school, I felt I was living the life of a double agent.

I went to class, did my homework, and hung out with Chloe. I quietly went through the daily installments of my existence. However, inside, my mind was in turmoil.

This test can save lives.

This test can end pancreatic cancer as we know it.

If this test had been around, maybe Uncle Ted would still be alive.

I had begun eating, drinking, and sleeping ISEF. I found myself mentally checking out during class while preparing my project speech over and over again in my head.

"Jack, any thoughts on the algorithm?"

"Uhhh."

"Jack, are you with us?"

"Sorry."

I floated through school in a daze until finally the morning came when my mom and I piled into our beat-up station wagon to set off on our journey to Pittsburgh. My dad and brother followed closely behind.

By the time we got into our hotel room it was late, but I could barely sleep. I kept playing and replaying all the different videos of ISEF award ceremonies from years past. The next morning, I woke up too excited to eat breakfast.

When I stepped into the convention hall, I felt the same rush I had as a seventh grader, tagging along with Luke. This was my dream. I headed straight for the registration booth.

Then . . . disaster struck. It all began with the simplest of questions.

"Could I see your identification, please?"

I knew that every competitor had to show a government ID to get into the conference. I checked my wallet. It wasn't there. I looked at my mom. She looked at me. Nothing. I had spent so much time focused on the actual event that I had completely forgotten the simple matter of getting through the front door.

"I forgot my ID," I said.

Despite my best pathetic help-me smile, the all-business ISEF worker remained unmoved.

"Sorry, there is just no way I can let you in without identification," she told us, her voice kind but stern. "It is policy."

I took a deep breath. There was no way I was turning back now. I knew there had to be *some* way to handle it. "Seriously," I pleaded. "I mean, are a lot of bad people really trying to sneak into a science competition?" I fake laughed. Her face was a rock.

For the next hour, which should have been spent preparing, I instead found myself pleading with the ISEF registration staff that I belonged. The all-business worker and another man disappeared behind a mysterious curtain for what felt like forever, and when the two finally reemerged they handed over my registration material.

"Good luck, Mr. Andraka."

As I put my official ISEF name tag on, I breathed a huge sigh of relief. For the first time, it all felt real.

Next, I was introduced to my fair coordinator, Valerie. All contestants were given a fair coordinator to guide them throughout the week. Valerie began giving me a tour, and showed me where to set up my display.

On the first day of the event, all the competitors are given a small cubicle-size space on the convention-room floor to showcase their experiments. The secret to a great display is to make sure it's both visually appealing and easy to understand. I used lots of colorful pictures and I broke my presentation down into different sections on methodology and data analysis. I included a part on the detection of mesothelin using antibodies too.

I felt confident, until I began to wander up and down the long rows of projects.

That person made a major breakthrough with Alzheimer's? How on earth am I going to top that?

That girl discovered a new protein cascade pathway. I don't even know what a protein cascade pathway is!

As I lay in bed that night, I mentally roamed the aisles of ISEF again, envisioning all the other projects and feeling less and less certain about my prospects. But when I woke the next morning, my optimism had returned. Day two was a free day for practicing our presentations and final inspections of our displays. As I rehearsed in front of my display, two kids, Bradley and Owen, wandered over to my booth to check out my project. They were both from New Jersey, and we hit it off right away. Later that night we all agreed to join up and go together to the pin exchange.

The ISEF pin exchange is kind of like the one they have at the Olympics where competitors from all around the world trade pins from their homelands. I brought a few dozen pins from Maryland, which had the shape of the state and an image of the Maryland flag, along with some Maryland-themed snow globes. I was able to trade for a Mexican sombrero and tons of interesting pins.

After the exchange, I was off with my new friends to the American Eagle Club, which Intel had rented out for the day to throw a giant party. You might think a dance with a bunch of science enthusiasts would be really lame. You would be wrong! The center of the dance floor was quickly turned into a giant mosh pit. In our delirious state, Bradley, Owen, and I decided it would be a fantastic idea to make balloon DNA hats to wear on our heads as we danced.

It was late when we left the dance floor and walked back to our rooms. We started talking about past ISEF winners, and Owen mentioned how in the videos he had watched, they always looked so restrained and straight-faced as they accepted their awards. Some of them didn't even smile!

"That's so ridiculous," I said. "These people are experiencing the greatest moments of their lives. They should show it!"

"If I won, I would cartwheel myself up to the stage," Owen said.

We all laughed. That night we made a promise to one another: if any one of us was fortunate enough to win any awards, he wouldn't hold back. It was just shy of three in the morning when I finally stumbled into my room, exhausted from dancing.

The next thing I remember was a pounding. At first I thought it was coming from inside my head, but it was the door.

"Jack, where are you? You are going to be late!" Valerie shouted through the door.

Oh crap!

It was the most important day of the competition—judging day. My body felt like it had been run over by a truck from lack of sleep and bobbing up and down on the dance floor for so long. As I tried to respond to Valerie, I realized I couldn't. I had lost my voice. I tried to tell her I was coming, but all that came out of my mouth was a bizarre, raspy croak.

A feeling of panic set in; while I had grown used to performing on little or no sleep, I didn't know sign language.

I opened the door and let her in. Unlike me, Valerie was super organized. She took one look at me and told me I needed electrolytes, immediately. She showed up two minutes later with three bottles of Gatorade.

"Drink," she ordered.

I sprinted to the convention floor, lugging the drinks, as fast as humanly possible. Once I was fully hydrated, my voice came back, and just in time.

Thank God for Valerie!

My favorite part of any science fair was presenting my idea. I came to learn that there is really no gimmick or trick, just a few basic guidelines.

Steady eye contact.

Wide, toothy smile.

Good posture.

Most important, there is no substitute for sincere passion. That's just something you can't fake. When the doors opened and a flood of people rushed the floor, I went straight to work.

"Hi, my name is Jack Andraka. I'm from Crownsville, Maryland,

and I'm fifteen years old. I'm a freshman in high school."

I reminded myself to be clear and concise. I imagined myself as a sort of carnival barker of science, where I sold my little stand of these important ideas to as many people as humanly possible.

"So basically what I've done here is create a paper sensor that can detect a wide array of diseases. Some notable examples include pancreatic cancer, ovarian cancer, and lung cancer. All these are life-threatening diseases where it's really crucial to detect them in their early stages, when survival rates are at their highest. I focused specifically on pancreatic cancer in this case because of its extremely low survival rates.

"So my paper sensor has single-walled carbon nanotubes, which are these atom-thick tubes of carbon, mixed with antibodies to this one cancer biomarker called mesothelin."

As I spoke, more and more people began to crowd around my small cubicle. I remembered from that time when I came with Luke that one of the goals was to get a big crowd of people in front of your stand. Once you get that first small group, that crowd tends to have a chain reaction that attracts even more people. And the more people around your stand, the more the judges took notice.

I continued: "When I compared it to the current gold standards of protein detection, my test was actually faster, over twenty-six thousand times less expensive, and over four hundred times more sensitive. And what I found was that my sensor, in a blind study, had a one hundred percent correct diagnosis of pancreatic cancer and could diagnose the cancer before it becomes invasive."

After I was done with my speech, I was ready for the questions. For this part, I never had to remind myself to smile; that part came easy!

I wasn't nervous. This was the culmination of countless hours of hard work, and I absolutely relished the opportunity to talk about my project. Sometimes standing for all those hours repeating the same things over and over again got repetitive, but the insightful questions always had a way of energizing me. I could feel the excitement bouncing off the audience. I began to take notice that several judges had crowded around my project, and both head judge chairs of the category had come over. That was a *very* good sign.

After the day was finished, the judging was over. The only thing left for me to do was wait for the results.

The next two days have separate award ceremonies. The first is for the special awards, which are given by scientific societies, organizations, and businesses, and the second day is for first- through fourth-place category awards, followed by the Best in Category, where the winners for each category go on to compete for the overall top prizes, including the Gordon E. Moore Award.

To build up the suspense, the fair organizers decided to place a six-hour public viewing session before the special awards ceremony. I worried about how I was going to stay hydrated without having the chance to go to the bathroom for six hours, but somehow I managed to pull it off. I was thrilled that there was always a throng of interested people hovering around my board.

The other contestants, as competitive as they were, had begun to take a liking to me too. They had given me the nickname "Cancer Paper Boy." I preferred this nickname to the many others I had received in middle school.

At the special awards ceremony, I found a few of my friends from math camp to sit with, but I was too nervous to say much. Waiting for the ceremony to start was agonizing. I knew it had been a big deal in my town when Luke won a special award. I wanted one too, and badly, but after seeing the competition, I told myself I needed to be prepared for disappointment. I mean, one kid had made a nuclear reactor!

During the announcement of the first few prizes, I won a special award for three thousand dollars! Remembering the promise I had made to Bradley and Owen, I let loose. I ran up to the presenter and gave a big, massive hug. I looked out into the audience. I wanted desperately to share the climax of my science fair career with my family. I saw my mom, tears in her eyes, clapping her hands together frantically. I ran into her open arms.

"Where are Dad and Luke?" I asked.

My mother's eyes flashed. I knew that look.

"They are late" was all she said.

I knew they were both going to get the full wrath of Jane Andraka's fury.

"I'm so sorry, Jack," she added.

It was okay, I thought. They might have missed my big moment, but we had it on tape and I'd play it again and again on the way home. Especially for Luke to see.

When my dad and brother finally arrived, my mother gave them the death glare of all death glares as I showed them my award. Amazingly, I wasn't through. Turns out my family would have more chances to share the moment with me. Throughout the night, I won multiple special awards, building a reputation for giving the presenters (including the strict-looking army sergeant) bear hugs and running around delirious with excitement.

I nearly passed out when I got called up for the prestigious Google Thinking Big Award, which is presented to the project that addresses a large and seemingly impossible problem. By that point, my mom was clapped out. I noticed that my dad kept putting his arm around me. He was thrilled, and proud, and very glad that my victory haul meant that my mom had temporarily forgotten that she was incredibly angry at him.

Finally, after a night of excitement, I stumbled out with an astounding six special awards, a number that tied with my hero Amy Chyao's ISEF record! I had won the most special awards of the night.

Now it was time for the announcement of the Best in Category winners. I looked at my other competitors in the field of medicine and saw my friend Owen from New Jersey, who had done ground-breaking research on Alzheimer's, and instantly thought, *It's him. He totally deserves it.*

But it was my name that was called. It was a huge honor in its own right, but it also meant that I was now in the running to compete for the biggest award of all—the Gordon E. Moore Award. The winner is selected not only on the basis of great research, but on the potential impact of the work as well—in the field of science and on the world at large.

When it was time for the grand finale, the highlight of the entire event, we all gathered together in a large auditorium. My category was one of the last to be announced, which meant I had to sit and watch for hours as, one by one, the winners took the stage. I was full of so much adrenaline that, at times, I had to repress the urge to scream randomly.

Finally, it was time. I straightened up in my seat, sitting very still. I could barely breathe. The presenter walked to the podium and began to speak.

"The second runner-up for the Gordon E. Moore Award is . . . Nicholas Schiefer." He was a seventeen-year-old from Canada who had a breakthrough in "microsearch," or the ability to search small amounts of information such as tweets or Facebook status updates, that would one day revolutionize how we access information. It was hard to comprehend how he had done it.

"The runner-up for the Gordon E. Moore Award is . . . Ari Dyckovsky." I couldn't believe he was second. I thought Ari's project was going to win. The eighteen-year-old from Virginia had found that once atoms are linked through a process called "entanglement," information from one atom will just appear in another atom when the quantum state of the first atom is destroyed. Using this method, organizations requiring high levels of data security, such as the National Security Administration, could send an encrypted message without running the risk of interception because the information would not travel to its new location; it would simply appear there.

Now I was confused. Who had beaten that kid? The two runners-up were now standing on the stage beaming, looking out at all the other students from the seventy different countries in the audience.

Of course, the kid who made the nuclear reactor. That's who won.

"The winner of the seventy-five-thousand-dollar 2012 Gordon E. Moore Award in . . .

"the category of . . .

"med . . ."

Medicine! That's me!

THAT'S ME!

I simply didn't have it inside me to wait for the award presenter to finish saying the words. My body just wouldn't allow it. I raised my arms and leaped straight out of my seat.

I ran up to the stage screaming and gasping for air.

I looked up at the giant television screen. There in big bold letters were three words: *Jack Thomas Andraka*!

That's me!!

I could see my picture in real time in front of me on the giant screen running up onto the stage.

I heard music and applause. I had to remind myself to breathe.

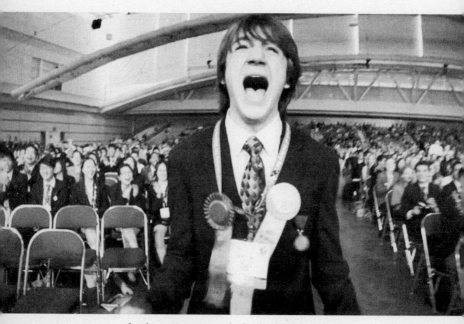

I rush onstage to receive the Gordon E. Moore Award.

After I got up on the stage, I fell to my knees and began bowing to the presenter. She laughed and tried to hand me the award. I got up and gave her the biggest embrace of all, lifting her off her feet.

I took the award in my hands and turned around to look out at the audience. I was screaming and I couldn't stop. From somewhere behind me confetti had exploded. Then came the announcement.

"And now, ladies and gentlemen, it is my honor to present to you the winner of the 2012 Intel Science and Engineering Competition."

Confetti rained down. I could make out individual faces in the audience. I could see my new friends from New Jersey and some of my friends from math camp. I could see my dad, who was tearing up, and my mom sitting next to him, beaming. Luke looked proud.

I was crying with my mouth open. As I stood on the stage, I remembered my long hours of work in the laboratory, the nights when it was just me and the Western blot, and the little stain I had left on the floor. I remembered what it was like to feel hated and bullied and rejected, but I also remembered Dr. Maitra, who decided to give me a chance. I thought of how much I loved my family, and how their support helped me shake off my blanket of depression and arrive at this moment. I thought of Uncle Ted, and how you can continue loving someone even after they are gone.

The weight of it all was almost too much to bear. Two years earlier no one would sit with me at lunch, but now within minutes of winning the award, I found myself being swarmed by kids I admired, asking for my autograph.

Congratulations, Jack!

How does it feel?

Can I have your autograph, Jack?

A middle-aged man emerged from the crowd. He wasn't a judge. He was a guest. Unlike the rest of the people gathered around me, he had a stern look on his face.

"I want to thank you," he said as he grabbed my hand.

"Thank me?" I said. "For what?"

There was a brief pause as I watched him tear up.

"Six years ago I lost the love of my life to pancreatic cancer," he said. There were tears coming down his cheeks now. "Looking at you, watching you talk . . . it makes me feel hopeful again."

I wrapped my arms around this total stranger in a warm embrace.

I told him about Uncle Ted, and how much he had meant to me.

"I'm sure he is proud of you," he said as he gave my hand one last squeeze before walking away.

After the festivities wrapped up, my family and I headed straight to the Potomac River to go kayaking. As I navigated through the rapids, I spent a lot of time reflecting on the week. A sudden rush of emotion swept through me as I realized that of all the great things that had happened to me, including the Gordon E. Moore Award, it was that stranger's words that had meant the most.

$$C_6H_8O_7 + 3NaHCO_3 \rightarrow 3CO_2 + 3H_2O + 3Na^+ + C_6H_5O_7^{3-}$$

Chapter 8

OH MY GOD, WE KILLED MORLEY SAFER

Seventy-two hours after winning the Gordon E. Moore Award, I finally got the chance to go through my phone, which had been buzzing for days. It was flooded with alerts. Most were messages from complete strangers on Facebook and Twitter who had Googled my name, found my account, and wanted to reach out and share in the excitement of the moment. The messages ranged from a simple "great job" to utter disbelief.

Did you really come up with a new way to prevent pancreatic cancer?

Is it true that you are really fifteen years old?

How did you do it?

At first, I tried to respond to every message, but as they kept arriving, I couldn't keep up. I also had other things on my mind: I needed to get ready to meet the press.

Typically the winner at ISEF had to fight to get any media coverage. I knew my hometown paper would interview me and write a nice article, as they did when Luke won a special award at ISEF, but generally the winners don't get very much attention.

We had just completed the drive back to Crownsville when we got a call for our first interview request—from CNN's *Early Start*. When my mom shared the news, I felt my knees get weak. The producers asked if they could fly my mom and me to New York City a day early to put us up at a luxury hotel. We didn't have to think too hard about that one.

The big interview was scheduled for May 23, less than a week after my winning the award. When we checked into the hotel, the staff at the front desk told us that everything we ordered would be paid for by CNN. Never ones to turn down a free meal, my mom and I happily feasted on room-service cheeseburgers.

The next day, we awoke to find a black car waiting outside to whisk us away to the CNN headquarters. We were met in the lobby and escorted to a room that was stocked with Krispy Kreme donuts, muffins, and the kind of small bottled drinks that cost way too much money for my family to ever consider purchasing.

"Who are these for?" I asked my mom.

We both looked around. We were the only ones in the room.

"Us, I think," she said.

I grabbed two gourmet chocolate milks and drank one after the other. I love chocolate milk. Unfortunately, I didn't think to bring my backpack or I would have taken a few more for the road. Before I could hit the glazed donuts, a producer wearing a futuristic headset walked over to let me know that makeup was ready.

I looked at my mom. She laughed at the look on my face. I followed the producer into a beauty salon–looking room, where he sat me in a chair and spun me around so I was staring at myself in the mirror. Next, a woman who looked like she was cut out of a fashion magazine came over and began caking my face with a thick powder that smelled faintly like sulfur. After my makeup was finished, I looked at my new rosy complexion and smiled. It was showtime.

As I walked onto the set, I worried that the lights were so bright and hot that they might mingle with my sweat and convert my makeup into cement, freezing my face in a perpetual expression of shock. The producer walked me over to a chair, and a second later I was introduced to the host, Alina Cho.

She took her seat directly across from me and began flipping through a packet of papers, reviewing some notes. A man behind the camera began a countdown—five, four—then at three he switched to hand signals—*two, one*—until pointing at us.

A green light came on the camera. After a brief introduction, we were live.

Alina hit me with her first question.

"Tell me, how did you come up with the idea? I know you were inspired by a close family friend."

I swallowed hard. The host was looking at me, smiling. My mom was behind me offstage. Now a camera was revolving around me in a 360-degree swivel. I felt nervous, but I had recited these lines so many times at the science fairs that I just sort of went into autopilot.

"So, after a close family friend passed from the disease, I became really interested in early detection of pancreatic cancer because early detection is one of the problems behind the huge death rate," I answered.

As soon as I began talking, I could feel all the nerves melt away. I was having fun. Next, she played a video of my reaction to winning the award.

"It is so remarkable," she said, laughing. "I watched it a couple of times."

It was a bizarre moment, akin to having an out-of-body experience; I was being interviewed on television while watching myself on a little television and being asked for my reaction, which was, of course, being televised. My mom was watching off to the side. My dad and brother were watching from home, along with hundreds of thousands of other viewers.

After Alina thanked me for coming in, it was all over. I felt both exhilarated by the experience and relieved that I didn't stumble. It also felt a little strange that after hours of travel, makeup, and antici-pation, the actual interview took only a few minutes. I was quickly escorted out of the studio. My mom ran up to me from where she had been watching.

"Jack, I'm so proud of you!" she said. "You did great!"

On the way home to Crownsville we could hardly contain our glee. The project had gotten the kind of national exposure we could only dream of. Now, we figured, it was time for me to turn the page and start thinking about the next project. We had barely unpacked our bags when the lady in charge of media relations for ISEF called. She sounded exasperated. Her office had been inundated with media requests.

"This is unprecedented," she said. "We aren't really sure how to handle it or what you want us to do."

"Well, that's okay. Jack's happy to talk to the press," my mom answered. "Just tell them yes. We can make time. How many requests have you received—a dozen? Twenty?"

There was a pause on the line.

"Thousands."

For once in our lives, my mom and I were speechless.

After all the frenzy of the past few weeks, it was time to get back to school. Between ISEF and the trip to Manhattan, I had missed nearly two full weeks.

I began my next morning with the same school-day routine. I woke up at five thirty, hopped in the shower for fifteen minutes, quickly made myself a few scrambled eggs, brushed my teeth, and by six thirty was sitting in the passenger seat of my dad's car for the thirty-minute car ride to school. I wasn't really sure how my teachers were going to react. Of course, I knew they would be okay with me going to ISEF, but the trip to New York could be a problem.

"I think I missed a biology test," I said to my dad.

"I think your teachers will let you make up any work you missed, Jack," he responded.

"I hope so."

I arrived in school as everyone was hitting their lockers. It was strange that nothing here had changed. I could hear shuffling as books were stuffed into bags, the metallic clang of lockers open- ing and closing, and the morning greetings as students passed each other in the halls. A few minutes before the morning bell, an announcement sounded over the loudspeaker.

"And congratulations to Jack Andraka, for winning the Gordon E. Moore Award."

In that singular instance, I felt my two worlds fuse. I hadn't been very social over the course of my freshman year and had barely spo- ken about my project. I chalked it up to residual walls that I still had up from my time in middle school. You don't get over that kind of ostracism and hatred quickly. Of course, I knew there was no way of hiding it after winning the regional science fair, but up until that moment, at least in my head, I had always kept the projects I was working on separate from my time in school. Now it felt as if my worlds had collided, and to my surprise, that felt okay.

As I walked through the halls, several classmates congratulated me. I slowed down as I passed by Damien's locker. For a moment we locked eyes. I hadn't seen him since the day he told me my project "sucked" at the regional fair. I smiled at him. He turned away, pretending he didn't see me.

The rest of the day went by like every other, except in Spanish class. When I walked in, I saw my teacher had brought me a big cake to celebrate my victory that said *"Felicitaciónes, Jack!"* I love cake. The whole class got to have a piece. Afterward, I went to speak with my biology teacher about letting me make up the test I had missed while in New York. She saw the worry on my face and broke out in laughter.

"Jack, are you serious? Of course!"

That was a relief. As a high school freshman, I wanted to do well in science.

As my freshman year drew to a close, I was expecting the media attention to end. But by June, the video of me winning the award had gone viral. What really blew my mind was that the majority of the interest was from the kind of kids who weren't exactly science geeks. In fact, many of them had never seemed to have much of an interest in science or math at all.

By the end of the second week of June, the phone in our living room was ringing off the hook with interview requests from different reporters, including those from some of my favorite magazines, like *Smithsonian*, *Discovery*, and *Popular Science*. Television crews from national news organizations like ABC World News and the BBC all wanted to talk to me.

"What is going on?" I asked my mom as she read down the list of requests.

"People look at you and see science as fun again," she said.

When we received a call from the news show *60 Minutes*, my mom couldn't say yes fast enough. Morley Safer, the legendary correspondent, had asked if he could come to my house to interview my family!

A few days later, Morley Safer arrived, flanked by a small army of camera-crew techs and assistants. As we all sat down, he began asking questions with the same famous voice I had heard so many times coming from my television on Sunday nights. My family and I took turns talking about our early family life, the things we liked to do, and, of course, our love for doing experiments in the basement.

"You do experiments in the basement?" Morley asked. "Can I see?"

My mom looked nervous. She had no idea what was down there.

"I think it's probably a real mess, right, boys?" she said.

She was looking at us for support. There was no way she wanted strangers, one of them being Morley Safer, seeing that part of her house. Luke and I didn't help my mom at all. Instead, we just sat there, acting like we hadn't heard her. Truth is, I hadn't been in the basement in a little while and wasn't exactly sure what it looked like—but I did know that one did not say no to Morley Safer, especially when Morley Safer was sitting across from you in your living room.

"Let's go check it out." He signaled to his camera crew, not waiting for an answer. We followed him down the narrow staircase to our basement lab.

The next thing we heard was a big thud, followed by a muffled groan. Morley Safer had tripped over some wires that were on the stairs. He had face-planted in my basement and he wasn't moving.

For a split second, everyone stood there frozen, looking down at the eighty-year-old television icon as he lay motionless on the Andraka family basement floor.

Oh my God, I thought. *We killed Morley Safer.*

His staff and my parents rushed over to help and that's when we saw a faint movement.

He's not dead!

"I'm okay," he said.

He didn't want any help. He insisted on pulling himself up and continuing with the interview as if nothing had happened.

After the *60 Minutes* segment aired, I noticed a snowball effect. The more times I appeared on television, the more other television reporters wanted to speak with me. Soon after the airing, we received an invitation to attend an event for the Clinton Global Initiative, a charitable foundation started by the Clintons. There was this big dinner filled with wealthy CEOs, a bunch of famous people I had never heard of, and of course, the Clintons themselves, who were the rock stars of the event.

The moment that former president Bill Clinton walked into the room, everyone was looking at him. He has a presence about him, as though he makes his own gravity.

He walked over to me and shook my hand.

"It's nice to meet you," he said. "You won the science award, right?"

Wow, it's nice for Bill Clinton to meet me?

"Congrats," he said.

My mom asked if she could take a picture and he happily agreed.

I made my way back to my seat, in shock over having just shook the hand of a former president, when I noticed that someone had moved my glass of Sprite. That's when Hillary Clinton approached me. She had this wide smile on her face. "Did I take your glass?" she asked.

This was awkward. She had, in fact, taken my glass, but I wasn't about to tell the secretary of state that she had swiped it from me.

"It's totally okay, no problem at all," I said in an apologetic tone.

She handed it back and pulled up a seat next to me.

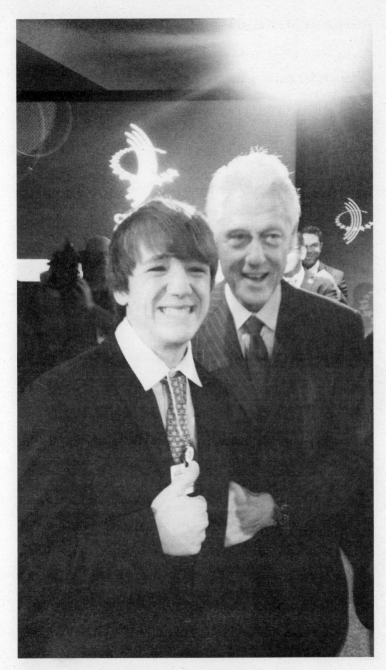

I meet Bill Clinton at a dinner for the Clinton Global Initiative.

"Tell me about yourself," she said.

By now, I'd told my story countless times to all kinds of different audiences, but this was a little bit different. As she listened, I was surprised by the warmth and care that she projected. At one point, while I was speaking, her daughter, Chelsea Clinton, walked by, touched my head, and said, "Nice hair."

After I told Hillary my story, I informed her that I didn't understand a lot about politics.

"Oh, it isn't as complicated as you might think. Did you ever see the movie *Mean Girls*?" she asked. "Well, politics is a lot like that movie," she continued. "Imagine all of these politicians as different cliques, and my job is to maneuver around them to get things done."

"Wow," I said. "In a way, high school never ends."

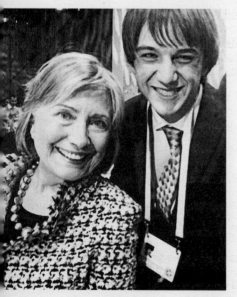

A selfie with Hillary Clinton!

She nodded. "Now you get it!"

Just when I didn't think it could get any more surreal, in October of my sophomore year, I was invited to appear as a guest on *The Colbert Report with Stephen Colbert*. I loved every second of being on *The Colbert Report*—even though I just sat there laughing through most of it. My favorite moment came when he asked me if I had ever considered using my powers for evil. I laughed so hard I couldn't talk.

I was struck by how different the real Colbert was when I got to speak to him for a few seconds off camera. He congratulated me on my accomplishments and asked me to keep it up, but he wasn't anything like his television persona. His tone was so serious and sincere.

However, my strangest post-victory moment by far came in November, after I was awarded the Sciacca Award in Research and Development and was invited to have an audience with Pope Francis. By now nothing seemed real, so, in that way, it all kind of made sense. When we arrived at the Vatican, my mom and I were escorted into a large ornate room where his staffers gave us a list of ground rules outlining things we could or could not do around the pope.

"You are not to touch any part of him for any reason," we were told, more in the tone of an interrogation than instruction. I could tell by the look on their faces that they were not kidding.

When Pope Francis finally emerged, he was dressed in his pope uniform with the big hat. He walked slowly and looked very frail. I kind of held my breath as he walked up to me, reminding myself not to shake his hand or go in for a hug. He stopped two feet away from my face, then, staring directly into my eyes, said words in a language that I couldn't understand. After he finished, he stared at me, waiting for a reaction. I didn't know what to do. I looked at my mom, who just wore this strained look on her face, as though she were trying to see something very far away. Then he did it again, this time in a different language. I smiled and nodded. Finally, on his fourth try, the words came out in English: "Congratulations on your award."

"Thank you very much," I said, holding my hands tightly together across my waist.

Back at home, I was receiving no special treatment. I still had to do the same normal chores, like keeping my room clean, taking the garbage out, and making sure our ferrets, Ginny Weasley and Phaedrus, were fed and bathed.

By now, my sophomore year of high school had morphed into a continuous blur of speaking appearances and interviews. My social life was virtually nonexistent. It seemed like most of my social interactions were with news reporters. I found myself answering the same questions again and again. I began to feel like a machine.

Yes, it feels great to get all this recognition.

No, I wasn't expecting to win the award.

Fortunately, my school had taken a real hands-off approach, basically assuring me that if I continued to do well on my tests, they wouldn't hold my lack of attendance against me. The few times I did show up to school, some of the teachers looked surprised to see me, thinking that I had dropped out.

However, the first few weeks of sophomore year, the talk of my high school wasn't about me, but about my brother, who was a senior at the time.

My mom received a call from the school secretary letting her know that she needed to come right away to deal with Luke. He had built an arc furnace in the school lab and his teachers had grown nervous when he mentioned that the device could heat up to one thousand degrees Fahrenheit. They grew even more nervous after he melted a steel screw to prove it. She raced to school to pick up Luke, along with his furnace. It soon found a spot among the collection of random projects in the Andraka family basement, just to the left of where we thought we had killed Morley Safer.

Most of the attention that I received during my sophomore year was positive. While the vast majority of people were supportive, there were some voices in the scientific community who doubted that my test worked, probably because they didn't think someone my age could make such a discovery. Some of my critics made me flash back to my time in middle school and seemed more focused on trying to tear me down on a personal level. One major publication even dedicated a thousand words to why they were NOT going to celebrate my accomplishments! There were times when I wanted to scream and shout or go online and respond to every single comment.

There were also attacks on my sexuality. I never really set out to become a gay role model, or to discuss my sexuality publicly. I wanted to share my ideas and to become a scientist. But being gay is part of who I am, so when it came up in an interview, I decided to be honest. I'd tried hiding before and that didn't work out so well for me. Besides, I remember going to fairs and participating in the science community for the first time and thinking, *Where are the people like me?* Maybe my story would make it easier for the next kid who wanted to come out. I tried to think about the messages I got from other gay teens when I got hate mail. And I got a lot of hate mail.

Fags burn in hell, you know that, right?

Most of the time I can tell by the subject line of the email that it's hate mail and I won't allow myself to open it, but sometimes my curiosity becomes my enemy.

If you ever change your sinful ways and decide you want to live a moral life, here is my email. It is never too late, Jack.

However, the hardest emails I get are from people who have lost someone to pancreatic cancer and want to know when they can get my test. Sadly, I have to tell people that it is going to take a while. My test still needs work. I need to refine it and also to publish my findings in a scientific journal where my work can be peer-reviewed. As Dr. Maitra says, the test is still in a preliminary stage. We need to examine patient samples to prove that in human serum, even when there are low levels of mesothelin, the test can still consistently detect cancer.

Then it needs to get approved by the Food and Drug Administration (FDA), the government agency responsible for protecting public health by ensuring the safety of most of the things we put into our bodies, including medicine and medical tests.

I've discovered that there is simply no quick way to push any-thing through the FDA. Receiving approval of even the simplest projects can take years and years, which can be especially hard if you happen to be one of the millions of people waiting for lifesav-ing treatments or drugs that are still pending. I've been told it will probably take another five or ten years for my test to hit the market. Knowing there was nothing I could do to speed this process, I tried to focus on giving interviews and speeches, and on what project I might work on next. In a recent interview Dr. Maitra said that he hopes I stay in biomedical science. I'm not sure where my next proj-ect will take me, but I feel so fortunate to have started in his lab. I know that he does not regret the day he took a chance on me, and I'm proud of that.

Halfway through my sophomore year, on February 11, 2013, I was at home packing to give a speech in London the next day. My dad was downstairs working out the bills.

I heard the phone ring, followed by the sound of my dad's voice.

"Jack, Jack, you better come down here," he said.

I ran downstairs.

"I just got off the phone with the White House," he said.

"The White House?"

Ohhhh! Luke's really *done it now,* I thought. This time his experi-ments were well beyond the letter-from-the-FBI stage. Now he had incurred the wrath of the president!

"You have been invited to the State of the Union address as a guest of the First Lady."

At first, I was confused—why would Michelle Obama want *me* to be *her* guest? I mean, I didn't even know her.

"Why?"

"Jack," my dad said in his you're-an-idiot voice. "To celebrate your accomplishments, of course."

"Oh my God! Oh my God! Oh my God!"

I ran around the kitchen, sliding around in my socks on the wooden floors.

"When do we need to leave?" I asked.

My dad, who had been standing there patiently watching me freak out, smiled.

"Jack, it's tomorrow."

I'm sure London will understand.

The next afternoon my mom, my dad, and I all piled into the family station wagon and set off on the fifty-mile drive to the nation's capital. Since I was allowed to bring only two guests, Luke had to stay home. That was my parents' call—sorry, Luke!

On the drive up, my dad had to endure me and my mom. First my mom got really excited, then her excitement got me excited, and our energies bounced off each other until words became screams and screams became squeals, until finally my dad, who is a wooden block of practicality, was on the verge of a mental breakdown.

When we arrived in Washington, we found a parking garage and walked the three blocks to our destination on Pennsylvania Avenue. We were greeted by a bunch of guys in very dark suits at the gate, some holding massive weapons.

My mom, who isn't intimidated by anyone or anything, stepped forward and did the talking for the rest of the family.

"This is Jack Andraka, he is here as a guest of First Lady Michelle Obama," she said proudly. "And we are Jack's guests."

The security officials looked down at me. I smiled and tried to look nonthreatening. My parents filled out some forms before another group of people in suits walked us across the lawn and into the White House. I knew that Uncle Ted would have gotten a real kick out of knowing that I was here because of him.

After opening the doors, we were deposited in this big dining room area, where we were allowed to mill around with a group of very important people who had also been invited for the speech.

In the room, I got to meet Tim

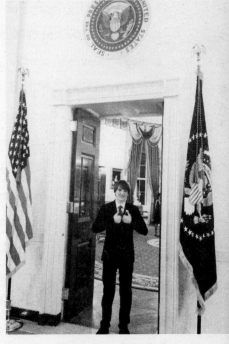

Striking a pose at the White House

Cook, the CEO of Apple. I recognized him right away and went up and introduced myself. He was very approachable, and after I told him my story, he shared that he had lost a close friend to pancreatic cancer. It wasn't until later that I realized he was talking about Steve Jobs.

I tried not to touch anything at the White House. From working at the laboratory, I had learned just how quickly one of my sneezes or stumbles could send things crashing to the floor. I spent my time pacing between these three huge, colored rooms: one painted blue, one red, and one white. Adorning the walls were fancy paintings of people I'm sure I should have known, but didn't. My attention was focused on the tuxedoed men walking around the room handing out plates of the most delicious steak skewers. I became addicted to them. I didn't feel comfortable taking two from the same tuxedo guy, so I tried to rotate among the different trays. I managed to eat seven skewers.

It was two hours later when a White House official walked us into a separate room, where we all got into a line to meet Michelle Obama and get pictures taken. The First Lady was so warm and friendly. She was hugging everyone in line and seemed genuinely happy to see all the people. In my head, I kept repeating my line to myself: *Thank you for inviting me.* As I approached, I saw one of her assistants whisper into her ear, telling her who I was.

"It's so great to meet you, Jack," she said.

"Thank you for inviting me," I said.

She gave me a big hug. I could feel her shoulder bones. She was incredibly strong.

"No, thank *you* for coming, Jack!"

We all posed for a picture together, along with Jill Biden. The First Lady thanked us again, and we were ushered away. A few minutes later I got to meet the First Dog, Bo. As I began to pet his head, he rolled on his back so I could scratch his tummy. I knew my dog, Casey, would be jealous when he smelled the First Dog on my hand.

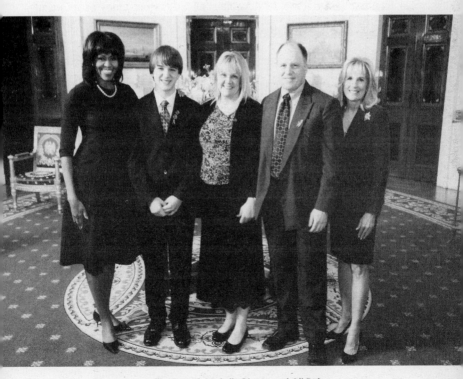

*My parents and I pose with Michelle Obama and Jill Biden
before the State of the Union address.*

Afterward we were divided into two groups. In the first group were the guests of the guests, who would see the speech in the White House movie theater. In the other group were the guests of the First Lady, who needed to be transported for the State of the Union address. I was shaking with excitement as I waved good-bye to my parents.

Once my group was piled into a car for the drive over to the Capitol, I noticed that agents on motorcycles were blocking traffic.

"Look," I said, finally breaking my silence to the group of very famous strangers. "They are shutting the streets down for us."

Everyone turned to look at me.

"Actually," a stern voice replied, "they aren't shutting down the roads for us. It's for the president."

What a party pooper.

After a short drive, we parked outside the Capitol and were shuffled into a secret entrance. An official led us up a set of stairs, and everyone was shown where they would be sitting on a chart. When it came time to show me where I would be sitting, the official pointed to the nearby stairwell. *How fitting!* I thought. I didn't care; I still had a view and I was just happy to be in the room.

I never felt so patriotic as when I heard the president announced. I stood up and clapped and cheered for him. Shortly after the State of the Union address began, a soft-voiced lady who looked like a librarian sat beside me on the stairs.

"You're a peasant too," I joked to her about our prestigious seating designation.

"I am," she responded, introducing herself as Valerie.

Valerie explained that she had been around the White House for a few years, and began sharing little tips and explaining to me what it was that I was watching.

"See, all the people standing to applaud are Democrats," she said. "Everyone sitting down is a Republican."

I jumped up and applauded every time President Obama mentioned innovation in science and medicine.

When the speech was over, my new friend Valerie asked me to follow her to a room off to the side. A second later, President Obama walked in. After seeing him as a talking head on television for so long, it was weird to see him standing in the flesh right in front of me. The president extended his First Hand to me and we shook hands. It was the softest hand I had ever touched.

"What was your project about, Jack?" he said.

Knowing he had more important things to do, I gave the leader of the free world the Cliffs Notes version of my science project.

He was surprisingly well versed in science. As I began to explain to him what nanotubes were, he stopped me.

"I know what nanotubes are," he said.

"What? No way!" I said.

"Yeah," he said, chuckling.

That moment talking with the president lasted less than two minutes, but it will stay with me for the rest of my life.

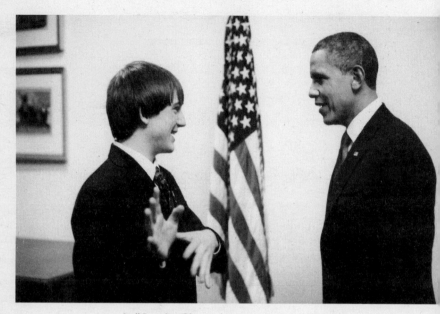

I tell President Obama about my pancreatic cancer test.

Days later, I was watching television when I saw my stairwell-sitting friend Valerie's face flash across the screen. That was the moment I realized that this super-warm lady who kept me company throughout the State of the Union was one of the most powerful people in the universe, White House Chief of Staff Valerie Jarrett.

Chapter 9

BREAKTHROUGH

As my sophomore year of high school continued on, I was feeling ready for my next project. In middle school, science was an escape from bullying and self-doubt, but now that I was older and more confident, I wanted to try something new just for the fun of it. I decided that I wanted to try to unlock the secrets of one piece of technology that has always fascinated me—the Raman spectrometer.

The Raman spectrometer is a machine that shoots a powerful laser that can break down almost any object on a chemical level. That means it can let us peel the layers back on everything from explosives to environmental contaminants. The problem is that because they are extremely delicate, as large as a small car, and cost up to $100,000, few people will get the benefits of this amazing technology.

I decided that if I could build a spectrometer that was smaller and less expensive, then it could be used for everyday tasks, like detecting pollutants in a stream or weapons in airplane luggage. I spent nine months working, before I finally had a breakthrough. I realized that if I could swap the Raman spectrometer's big laser for a laser pointer and its liquid nitrogen–cooled photodetector (which it uses to determine the chemical makeup of whatever material is being analyzed) with an iPhone camera, I could reduce the cost to fifteen dollars and make it the size of a smartphone. My spectrometer is 7,000 times less expensive and 1,250 times smaller, while also being just as efficient! This project was very different from working on my pancreatic cancer test, because I had to learn a lot about engineering. Some of the vocabulary was confusing.

But once I figured it out, I had a new project, which I called "The Tricorder: A Novel Raman Spectrometer for Real World Applications." I entered it into the Anne Arundel County Regional Science and Engineering Fair and was rewarded for my efforts with a first-place prize and another trip to ISEF, this time in Phoenix, Arizona.

When I got to ISEF, I found myself in the unfamiliar position of being admired by the other contestants. Throughout the event, students kept coming up to me, asking if they could take a picture with me. I was flattered, but while I enjoyed the limelight, I didn't spend nearly enough time practicing my presentation. I also knew this year's project wasn't quite as great as last year's.

My favorite project belonged to Ionut Budisteanu. The

nineteen-year-old from Romania was awarded first place for using artificial intelligence to create a four-thousand-dollar self-driving car with 3D radar and mounted cameras that could detect traffic lanes and curbs, along with the real-time position of the car. Wow, did he deserve to win! I felt fortunate when I won two special awards.

Watching Ionut standing on the stage holding the Gordon E. Moore Award brought back a lot of memories of the best moment of my life. It was hard to believe it had been three whole years since Uncle Ted had passed and one year since I had run screaming up to the stage to accept my award.

I found that, over the course of time, Uncle Ted's words had hardened into memorials that served as guideposts in my mind whenever I felt like I was at a crossroads.

I'd stopped expecting to see Uncle Ted's beat-up car come down my driveway for a day of crabbing, but I hadn't forgotten his voice. I could hear him urging me on in the moments when I wanted to quit, or the times when I received a particularly hurtful email. Uncle Ted made the moments of his life count by making a positive impact on the world. I wanted to do the same.

During my junior year, Chloe and I were walking around the Baltimore Harbor one day, being totally grossed out by all the disgusting water bottles bobbing in the water. I thought, what if we could create a water bottle that could purify water? Chloe and I began bouncing ideas off each other and formulating a plan of action.

"It would need to be a water bottle that people used again and again, with a filter unlike anything on the market today," she said.

"That would take a biosensor that would detect anything that might be harmful," I added.

"It would have to be inexpensive," said Chloe, "so that it could reach people in third-world countries where contaminated drinking water is such a killer."

Chloe and I had become even closer. We liked to watch the Iron Man movies together, and were particularly interested in the lab in Tony Stark's house and all the gadgets he had. But Chloe was also incredibly smart, and together we were like a scientific odd couple. We were both minorities in the science world, me for being a gay kid, and her for being a black girl.

We got right to work on our filter. To accomplish our goal of creating a purifying water bottle, we had to figure out how to produce microfluidic structures, or devices that deal with volumes of fluid on the order of tiny measurements of water known as nanoliters. To do this, we had to come up with an entirely new procedure and custom-make our own equipment. It took six months of research, trial and error, and hard work to create a microfluidic biosensor to detect the presence of chemicals.

I knew from my previous experiences that if we just kept at it, we would get where we wanted to be. By working together, we created a plastic filter made from recycled plastic water bottles. We attached amino acids to these bottles, which work like magnets to attract out all the dangerous contaminates like mercury and pesticides. The filter we made is able to monitor water contaminants rapidly, inexpensively, and easily.

Our filtration system can be used in third-world countries, where dirty drinking water takes countless lives each year, and it has other uses, like improving the effects of fracking, oil spills, and even chemical spills. Chloe and I entered our project in the Siemens We Can Change the World Challenge, a nationwide contest that has become the biggest environmental sustainability competition. To compete, students have to identify an environmental issue that has global impact and provide a viable, replicable solution. Chloe and I won first place and got to share fifty thousand dollars in scholarship money! Winning with my best friend, my scientist partner in crime, was the best.

I still miss a lot of school these days because I travel and

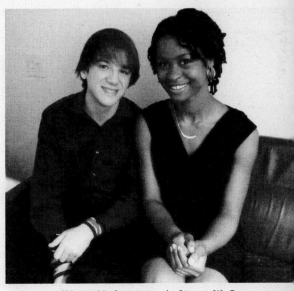

Chloe and I after winning the Siemens We Can Change the World Challenge

give lots of speeches. For the most part, I love all the exposure and attention I've received since winning the Gordon E. Moore Award. Sometimes I still don't understand what a teen science geek is doing meeting the president or the pope. However, I like it best when I'm by myself in my basement, digging into my next project.

One day, while I was sitting in my AP Chemistry class junior year, I had another idea. We were learning about equilibrium, which was boring me to tears, so I skipped ahead to another chapter about a process called photocatalysm, which is when organic chemicals are broken down using light. I began to wonder if I could create a paint that could break down different air contaminants that are harmful to breathe. After all, most people spend, like, 90 percent of their time indoors, and breathing stale air is not good for your health, especially if you have asthma or some other respiratory problem. I'm still working on this project, but I'm hoping that I can make a paint that is cheap and comes in nice colors.

I'm also hoping that my pancreatic cancer detection test can be modified to detect other diseases. Since almost every major disease has proteins that show up early and can be used as biomarkers, by switching out mesothelin antibodies and using an antibody for another target protein, I'm hoping my test can detect diseases such as Alzheimer's, HIV, or even heart disease to give doctors a head start on treatment.

I've even thought about combining my paper test strip with my modified Raman spectrometer. That way, by using a little device the size of a phone, people could screen themselves at home for different diseases. This would help doctors catch problems even earlier, and it would seriously cut down on hospital wait times.

Right now there's an exciting change going on in how we detect different illnesses. The old way of doing things, by scanning and poking and taking temperatures, is giving way to a new method called molecular diagnostics, which focuses on the proteins in your blood. This means that certain diseases can be caught before a patient feels sick or has any symptoms.

These days, it seems like everywhere I look there is something exciting going on in the world of science and technology. Did you know that telekinesis, or the ability to move things with the power of your mind, is actually a real thing? Using a new technique called electroencephalography, five students from the University of Minnesota College of Science and Engineering were able to harness their brain waves to control the motion of a helicopter!

Or did you know that the Palm Islands were built up out of the ocean by engineers in Dubai and made in the shape of palm trees?

With all the breakthroughs in science and technology happening everywhere, sometimes I just don't understand why other people my age aren't more interested. I still remember back in elementary school when my classmates seemed to love science as much as I did. I lived for getting my hands dirty, taking things apart, and figuring out how the world worked. I remember watching caterpillars turn into butterflies in class, and learning for the first time what happens when you put an Alka-Seltzer into a bottle of Coke.

But then something changed for a lot of my classmates. I noticed that many of them became uninterested in science. The wonder was gone. Some even began to hate science, and math, too. I don't exactly know why this is. Maybe it just wasn't cool anymore, or it was easier to spend time on your phone or playing video games.

I'm optimistic though. I spend a lot of time going to different events and talking about STEM education reform. STEM stands for science, technology, engineering, and math. Last summer, President Obama announced a new campaign to train one hundred thousand STEM teachers, with the goal of providing STEM learning opportunities for eighteen thousand low-income students and inspiring more kids to become involved.

I have lots of ideas for changing the way school is set up. I want school to be less like sitting and memorizing facts from a textbook and more like working in my basement. I want there to be open access so that everyone, no matter how old you are or how much money you have, can read about the amazing research that takes place every day. I never would have made my discoveries if I hadn't been able to read articles online, and many of those I had to pay for. I want them to be free so a kid in rural India has as much of a chance as I do at discovering the world's next breakthrough.

Today I've been sitting down at my kitchen counter, trying to work. It hasn't been easy. The last few hours have been one distraction after another. The biggest problem, at the moment, is Luke, who is home from Virginia Tech, where he is studying engineering. He won't shut up about a pizza he is making, and he knows that I can't leave the kitchen because it's the only place in the house that has Wi-Fi at the moment.

Now he has left the room but is making bird noises from the family room. He is seriously so annoying.

There is also something else on my mind. Recently, I was on a

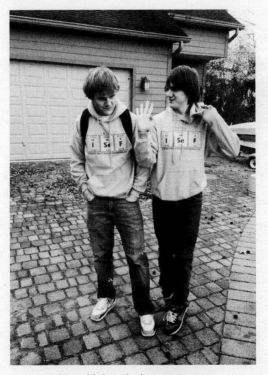

*Me and Luke in the driveway wearing
our matching ISEF sweatshirts*

trip back from a conference in London, watching the movie *Wall-E*, about an intelligent robot.

I can't help but wonder: What if I could find a way to make robots really small and smart so they could swim through the bloodstream and treat medical conditions?

To make this work, these robots would have to be nanobots. Nanorobotics is the creation of robots so small, they have to be measured in nanometers, which are one-billionth of a meter long. I'd have to learn a lot more about nanobots. I also don't know a lot about the human circulatory system, but I know some great research sites online that will help me with that.

If this is going to work, these little robots won't just have to be small, they will also have to be agile enough to navigate through the circulatory system.

What if I could make a robot flexible? How would I do that? If anyone has any ideas, please let me know. After all, I'm waiting to hear about your projects next. In the meantime, I'm going to get to work.

#BREAKTHROUGH

If you're tired of hearing our generation getting trashed all the time as a group of self-entitled slackers, it's up to each one of us to break through and change that perception.

What is the one thing you can do to change the world? Share your own inspirational photos or actions with #Breakthrough.

ACKNOWLEDGMENTS

There are *so* many amazing people I'd like to thank, without whose help this book would not have been possible!

My literary managers, Sharlene Martin and Clelia Gore of Martin Literary and Media Management, who not only did an amazing job representing me, but have become my friends. You both are so awesome! Thank you! I'm especially grateful for all the amazing food you all fed me when we hung out in New York City.

To Matthew Lysiak, for his tireless work in helping me with this manuscript.

I was blown away by *everyone* at HarperCollins, who had faith that a book by a science geek could inspire others!

To my editors, Nancy Inteli and Olivia Swomley, who did a fantastic job of guiding this book and pushing me to go deeper.

This book would also not have been possible without the help and support of the awe-inspiring team of professionals at Harper-Collins: Lisa Sharkey, Emily Brenner, Andrea Pappenheimer, Diane Naughton, Sandee Roston, Matthew Schweitzer, Julie Eckstein, Cindy Hamilton, Victor Hendrickson, Laura Raps, and the entire legal team.

I want to thank my mom, Jane Andraka, and my father, Steve Andraka, for not murdering me or sending me to reform school after any one of those number of times when I almost blew our house up or set loose strange bacteria in the kitchen. You both are the best parents ever. Ever. Thank you!

And before he walks upstairs and punches me in the face, I better thank my older brother, Luke. He is actually a pretty cool guy and one of a small handful of people who gave me support when I needed it most.

Luke, you are one of my best friends. Thank you!

THE SCHOOL OF JACK
EXPERIMENTS, TIPS, AND FACTS

F	Ne
Cl	Ar
Br	Kr
I	Xe
At	Rn
Uus	Uuo

Yb	Lu
No	Lr

$$C_6H_8O_7 + 3NaHCO_3 \rightarrow$$

$$3CO_2 + 3H_2O + 3Na^{+1} + C$$

H											
Li	Be										
Na	Mg										
K	Ca	Sc	Ti	V	Cr	Mn	Fe	Co	Ni	Cu	Zn
Rb	Sr	Y	Zr	Nb	Mo	Tc	Ru	Rh	Pd	Ag	Cd
Cs	Ba	*	Hf	Ta	W	Re	Os	Ir	Pt	Au	Hg
Fr	Ra	**	Rf	Db	Sg	Bh	Hs	Mt	Ds	Rg	Cn

EXPERIMENTS

I believe learning is something you *do*. You don't need to be officially enrolled in school to make a difference in your life and your education. In the spirit of discovery, I've included ten experiments for you to try. Be sure to obey the Andraka family rule: Don't blow up the house! You should also get permission from an adult before trying these.

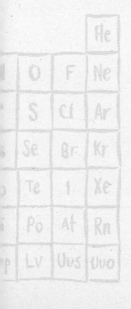

EXPERIMENT #1
Make Your Own Lava Lamp

Remember when Lava Lamps were cool in the sixties? Yeah, neither do I. But even if you're not a flower child from that era, you are going to absolutely *love* this experiment. This experiment shows a colorful way to explain the powers of two of my favorite things, sodium bicarbonate and citric acid.

Materials

- A vase or large glass water bottle (anywhere from 20 ounces to 2 liters)
- Food coloring (the more colors the better!)
- Store brand Alka-Seltzer
- Vegetable oil
- Grateful Dead music (this is entirely optional)

NOTE: Read carefully, this is very important—under no circumstances should you use an antique glass vase that has been in your family for generations. Especially if it is one that was handed down from your beloved aunt Ida. Seriously, don't do it! Just ask your parents to help get you one.

Procedure

1. Fill the vase or glass bottle about three-quarters of the way full with the vegetable oil.

2. Add about half a cup of water or fill until there is only an inch or two of space left at the top of your vase or bottle.

3. Begin adding drops of the food coloring, about six to seven drops, depending on the size of your vase or bottle. I like to use a bunch of different colors, but any amount or color works. Keep adding the drops until your water is filled with color.

4. Cut the Alka-Seltzer tablets into quarters and drop one of the quarters into the water.

5. Now wait for it . . . wait for it . . . wait for it . . . BUBBLES!!

6. Tap "play" on the Grateful Dead music (again, this part is optional) to bring home the full effect of the time warp.

7. After a few minutes, when the bubbles begin to slow down, you can add another quarter piece of Alka-Seltzer for a quick recharge.

8. Now it's time to get creative. Try throwing sugar, salt, or even Goldfish crackers into the water and see the different reactions.

Discussion

This experiment is a fun way to demonstrate how sodium bicarbonate and citric acid (the two main ingredients in Alka-Seltzer) react.

When the tablet hits the water and begins to dissolve, all the ingredients mix together and carbon dioxide is released in the form of bubbles rising to the top. The bubbles work to mix the oil and colored water (and remember, water and oil prefer to stay apart from each other).

Now sit back and behold the hypnotizing powers of the Lava Lamp. Move it around in your hand and watch as the liquid gels and separates into different shapes and colors.

Meditate on the wonders of the universe! And the wonders of sodium bicarbonate!

And please . . . turn that hippie music off.

EXPERIMENT #2
The Incredible Bendable Rubber Bone

One of the cool things that I have always loved about science is how it can be used to amaze and astound friends and family members. After all, most magic tricks are really science. If you ever want to see a real magician at work, find a world-class physicist.

In this experiment, we are going to take an everyday object that you thought you knew and, using the powers of science, zap it of its strength.

Materials

- A large glass jar
- A bottle of vinegar
- A chicken drumstick

Procedure

1. The first order of business is to eat a great big chicken dinner. Now grab a drumstick, or leg bone, and eat all the meat off it. If you are anything like me, that shouldn't be a problem.

2. After you finish eating your dinner and washing it down with a tall glass of milk, take the leg bone and rinse it off in

water. Now gently try to bend the bone. It should be hard and unbendable.

3. Put the bone into your jar and pour your vinegar over it. You don't need to fill the whole jar; just make sure the bone is soaked. Now put the lid on the jar, stick it somewhere up on a shelf, and forget about it for the next three days.

4. After the three days are up, carefully take your bone out of the jar and rinse it off. WARNING: When you open your jar you might be overwhelmed by a pungent odor. That's the vinegar. It won't hurt you, but it might make you feel like throwing up that chicken dinner you ate three nights earlier.

5. Now that you've survived the smell, notice how different the bone feels in your hand. Try bending it again. This time, instead of feeling hard, it should bend like a piece of rubber.

Discussion

Remember in *Batman* when the Joker fell into the vat of acid and his face melted? Just like the liquid that messed up the Joker's face, vinegar is an acid, although a much weaker type, but it can do just as much damage if given the opportunity. That's because what gives chicken bones (and the bones inside your body) their superior strength is calcium. Calcium, or Ca, is an amazing chemical element needed for all living organisms, and is used in mineralization (the way our cells soak in the minerals to help harden them) of bone, teeth, and shells.

However, it isn't without its weaknesses. In the case of calcium, vinegar happens to be its Kryptonite. While you were playing video games the last three days, the vinegar was working hard to strip the calcium out of the bone. Taking the calcium out of a bone is kind of like pulling out the stake from a scarecrow. All that is left is the soft bone tissue, leaving nothing to keep the bone hard. This experiment is also fun to try with an egg—the vinegar will completely dissolve the shell, leaving you with a see-through egg!

EXPERIMENT #3
Make Your Own Rock Candy

With all that talk of chicken dinner, maybe it's time for dessert? This experiment is the perfect excuse to consume vast amounts of colored sugar by making a supersaturated solution.

Materials

- A clothespin or piece of string
- One cup of water
- Two wooden chopsticks
- Three cups of sugar
- A tall narrow glass
- A medium-size pan

Procedure

1. Take one chopstick and lay it across the top of your glass. Take the second chopstick and clip it to the first one using the clothespin, or tie them together using string. Position the chopsticks so that one is hanging straight down into the glass, without touching the sides or bottom. Put the glass off to the side.

2. Pour the cup of water into the medium-size pan and heat.

When the water reaches a boil, begin adding the sugar, one quarter of a cup at a time. Stir until the sugar dissolves before adding more. You will notice that it becomes harder to dissolve the sugar as you add more and more. Be careful not to burn yourself!

3. When you've added all the sugar, turn the heat off, grab some pot holders, and remove your pan of boiling sugar water from the stove. Set it aside someplace where it can cool and leave it alone for at least twenty minutes.

4. After it's cooled, add some food coloring. Make sure you add enough coloring to make the water dark, as the color will fade quite a bit.

5. Take your jar and remove the chopsticks. Carefully pour in the sugar solution until there is just a little room at the top. Now put your wooden chopsticks back into the glass, making sure that one is hanging straight down into the water without touching the sides.

6. Find a nice quiet spot where you can leave your jar where it will not be disturbed by that curious cat of yours. Now you will need to wait between three and seven days.

7. While you are waiting, you can look, but don't touch. It's fun to watch your sugar crystals as they grow.

8. When the crystals have formed along the stick, take your chopstick out of the glass and eat your rock candy!

Discussion

This experiment works because boiling water can hold the sugar only when both are very hot. As the water cool and evaporates, small crystals of sugar will encrust the chopstick and sometimes the glass. These tiny seed crystals provide starting points for larger crystals.

The crystals grow because the supersaturated solution is unstable—it contains more sugar than can stay in a liquid form—so the sugar will come out of the solution, in a method called precipitation. Then, as time passes and the water evaporates, the solution becomes even more saturated and sugar molecules will continue to come out of the solution and collect on the seed crystals on your chopstick. The rock candy crystals grow molecule by molecule. Your finished rock candy will be made up of about a quadrillion molecules attached to your stick.

Did you know that rock candy is one of the oldest forms of candy and was originally used by pharmacists to make medicines? You can tell your parents that when they are giving you grief for eating so much sugar.

EXPERIMENT #4
The Mighty Unbreakable Bubble

Remember Glinda the Good Witch from *The Wizard of Oz*, who cruised around all over Munchkinland in that hovering magical bubble thing? Well, with this experiment, we will use the power of science to finally pull the curtain back to reveal the magic behind the mighty unbreakable bubble.

Materials

- Two tablespoons dish soap
- One cup of distilled water
- Cotton gloves
- A bottle of bubbles (you know, the one with the little wand that you can get at your local supermarket)
- One tablespoon corn syrup (check the syrup section at your local grocery store)
- A mixing bowl

Procedure

1. Pour the cup of distilled water into the mixing bowl.
2. Add two tablespoons of dish soap and one tablespoon of Karo syrup and stir until everything is mixed up.

3. Slip on your cotton gloves, take the magic bubble wand out of your bubble container, dip it into your soapy mix, and begin blowing bubbles. The goal is to make really huge bubbles.

4. These are no ordinary bubbles. See how you can gently catch the bubbles and tap them up or down with your gloved hand? Watch them bounce off the glove and back into the air!

TIP: This experiment works best on humid days when there is a lot of moisture in the air and the walls of the bubble have more support. Experiment to figure out what materials make the bubbles bounce the best. Try your knee or hat. Or even your annoying brother's or sister's head!

Discussion

In normal bubbles, the soapy mixture on the outside is actually made of three layers: soap, water, and another layer of soap.

What causes these normal bubbles to pop so easily is that, over time, the water that is trapped between the layers of soap evaporates and the force of gravity causes the superthin walls, which can measure as little as a millionth of an inch, to collapse.

And that's only if you are lucky enough that a bubble's other worst enemies—dirt and oil—don't get to it first.

The reason our unbreakable bubble will bounce off a surface that would normally cause it to break is because the corn syrup found in the Karo gave it an extra layer of support, making it thicker. This thicker wall keeps the water inside from evaporating as quickly, which gives the bubble its impressive staying power. Wearing the gloves helps out by safeguarding against dirt and oil.

EXPERIMENT #5
Dr. Jekyll and Mr. Milk

One of the things that has always fascinated me about science is how it can take all these seemingly boring, ordinary, everyday items and reveal a deep, explosive underbelly that was hiding beneath the surface.

In the Dr. Jekyll and Mr. Milk experiment, we will take our well-known morning cereal companion and then, through the powers of science, make an amazing display of colors by adding one simple ingredient—dish soap.

Materials

- A large dinner plate
- Milk (whole or 2 percent)
- Cotton swabs
- Dish soap
- Food coloring (red, yellow, green, and blue)

Procedure

1. Pour milk onto your dinner plate until the bottom is completely covered, but not so much that it spills over onto the table.

2. Give the milk a few seconds to settle.

3. Add one drop of each of your four colors of food coloring to the center of your milky plate (the order of the colors is up to you and doesn't really matter).

4. Take just a single drop of your dish soap and drip it onto the end of the cotton swab. Gently dip the soapy end of the cotton swab in the middle of the milk. Now hold it there for twenty seconds and watch the amazing display of color.

Discussion

This experiment is all about the violent clash between the milk and the dish soap. The milk contains vitamins, minerals, proteins, and, most important (at least for our experiment), tiny droplets of fat.

If you have read *The Strange Case of Dr. Jekyll and Mr. Hyde*, you know that those names apply to polar-opposite personalities trapped inside the same person.

Dish soap has similar "bipolar" characteristics (remember, *bi* means two). The soap has one personality, or characteristic, that is hydrophilic, meaning it *loves* water. In fact, it loves it so much it melts right into it and dissolves.

Then there is the other side of dish soap, its inner Mr. Hyde, that absolutely despises water. It's hydrophobic, or water-fearing, and is so freaked out by the water that it desperately latches on to the fat in the milk, in a violent, thrashing sort of way. It is this reaction that makes this experiment so cool.

Did you ever hear lifeguards talk about the danger of trying to save someone who is drowning? That's because the drowning victim can become so full of adrenaline that they might actually pull even an accomplished swimmer down with them.

The same principle is at work in our pan of milk. The soap is so afraid of water that it scrambles to grab onto any piece of fat it can find, and once there, it holds on and contorts the fat in all kinds of crazy directions. The only role of the food coloring is to make this spastic interaction visible.

After a few minutes, the soap will become evenly mixed with the milk and the action will slow down until it eventually stops.

TIP: Experiment by dabbing your soapy cotton swab at different places in the milk. What happens? Also, how does it change when you switch from whole milk to 2 percent?

And one quick word of warning: Remember, no matter how thirsty you might become, milk that has soap and food coloring in it might look delicious, but drinking it will cause you to gag. Seriously.

EXPERIMENT #6
It's Potato O'Clock!

Have you ever *really* needed to know the time, but when you looked all you could find were potatoes?

We are all aware of the many purposes of the potato—mainly, to be next to our cheeseburger and slightly to the left of our pickle—but did you know that if you are in a pinch you can use your potato as a battery?

Materials (check your local hardware store)

- Two ten-centimeter lengths of thick copper ground wire
- Two large galvanized zinc nails
- Three alligator-clip wires
- Two fresh potatoes
- A simple low-voltage LED clock that functions from a one-to two-volt button-type battery

Procedure

1. First, open the clock's battery compartment and remove the button battery.
2. Look inside and find the two battery connections. One should be marked with a plus sign and the other with a

minus sign. That is where you will be hooking up your potato.

3. Take your first potato and poke one end of your copper wire inside it at least half an inch. Now find a place as far away from the wire as possible to stick your nail into the potato. You don't want them to touch! I'll explain why later.

4. Repeat step 3 with potato two, inserting the copper wire and nail—again, as far from each other as possible.

5. Now use one alligator-clip wire to connect the copper wire of your first potato to the plus connection in the clock.

6. Grab another alligator-clip wire and, this time, use it to connect the zinc nail of your second potato to the negative connection in the clock.

7. Then take your third alligator-clip wire and use it to connect the zinc nail of your first potato to the copper wire of your second potato.

8. Now look at that! Your clock is running on nothing but the magic of the mighty spud!

Discussion

Congratulations! You just made an electrochemical battery, also known as an electrochemical cell. In other words, with the power of the potatoes, you were able to convert chemical energy to electric energy by inspiring something called a spontaneous electron transfer.

In the case of the potatoes, our favorite starch acts as a kind of buffer between the power from the zinc in the nail and the copper wire. The juice from the potato helps transfer the electrons over the copper wires of the circuit, which channels the energy into the clock. If your potatoes are fresh enough, you can actually run your clock on potato power for months!

NOTE: If the zinc and the copper touched inside of the potato, they would still react, but they would only generate heat.

Your friends may be chuckling at your potato clock today, but just wait until that zombie apocalypse hits, there is a shortage of batteries, and you are the only one who is able to tell time—we will see who is laughing at your amazing potato clock then!

EXPERIMENT #7
The Sucking Glass

Have you ever wondered if science sucks? The answer is . . . sometimes. Using only simple household items, you will create your very own vacuum, capable of sucking up water.

Materials

- A drinking glass or other clear glass container
- A ceramic plate
- A candle (make sure your candle fits inside the glass)
- Food coloring
- Matches
- Water

Procedure

1. Pour water onto your plate until the bottom is covered.
2. Add a few drops of food coloring to the water and mix until the color is evenly distributed.
3. Put the candle in the middle of the plate and ask a parent to light it.
4. After waiting at least a few seconds, place your glass upside down over the candle so it is completely covered.
5. Watch what happens when the candle goes out . . .

Discussion

Once the cup is covering the candle, the flame will eventually run out of oxygen and go out. While the candle was burning, it was heating the air inside the glass, and heated air expands. You may even notice some bubbles escaping from the bottom of the glass. But when the flame has gone out, the air begins to cool down, and cool air contracts. This contraction is what pulls the water from the plate into the glass.

EXPERIMENT #8
The Mad Scientist

Have you ever suspected that something dark and mysterious has been growing where your brother throws his disgusting dirty socks even though everyone has reminded him that his laundry basket is only a few feet away?

Now with the Mad Scientist experiment we finally have the tools to prove your suspicions.

Materials

- A petri dish of agar, a gelatinous substance made from seaweed that bacteria love to eat (if you search online, you should find some for under ten dollars. You can also use agar powder. Just add water or fruit juice to make a gel.)
- A few sheets of old newspaper
- A cotton swab
- A disgusting surface

Procedure

1. Grab the cotton swab and find a surface in your house that warrants further investigation. I always like to pick the most disgusting surface I can find. Take your cotton swab and

gently rub it a few times against the surface you choose.

2. Rub the swab over the agar a few times, then close the lid and seal up the petri dish. Be sure not to open the dish again, as you don't want the bacteria getting out. Also, make sure you throw away the used cotton swabs.

3. Now find a warm area where your petri dish won't be disturbed and let it sit for two to three days.

4. It won't be long before those tiny invisible bacteria will grow large enough to be visible to the naked eye. Soon you should see a whole bunch of new life growing.

5. It helps to write down your observations from day to day or take cell phone shots so you can remember the changes.

6. You can repeat the experiment by swabbing all kinds of surfaces. If you really want a scare, try under your fingernails. You wouldn't believe what creatures have been living rent-free under there!

NOTE: When finished, carefully get rid of the bacteria by wrapping up the petri dish in old newspaper before throwing it in the trash. Remember, don't open the lid of the dish—you don't want the bacteria you've been growing anywhere near you!

Discussion

Now that you've seen what is living in your brother's room, you might feel the impulse to call a hazmat crew or the Centers for Disease Control. Don't do it! At least not yet.

With the agar plate and a warm climate, we provide the perfect environment for the bacteria to grow. If you watch long enough, eventually they will grow into individual colonies, each cloning the original.

The truth is that while, yes, your brother needs to work on his hygiene, bacteria are everywhere.

Bacteria are a member of a large group of unicellular microorganisms that have cell walls but are missing an organized nucleus. A gram of soil typically contains about forty million bacterial cells. A milliliter of fresh water usually holds about one million bacterial cells. Our planet is estimated to hold at least five nonillion bacteria. Get the point? Bacteria are *everywhere*!

Don't freak out! Our immune system usually does a great job of making sure these bacteria are harmless. That isn't to say that your brother's room shouldn't still be condemned as a toxic waste site.

EXPERIMENT #9
How to Make a Rain Cloud in a Bottle

Have you ever looked at your smug sibling after he just spent an hour and a half in front of the mirror making his hair oh so perfect and wished you could make a rain cloud burst open above his head at just the right time?

Well, check out this really cool experiment where you can make your own real rain cloud in a bottle!

Materials

- A plastic water bottle with a sports cap that pops open and shut
- Matches
- Warm water

Procedure

1. Pour about an eighth of a cup of warm water into your plastic water bottle.
2. Put the cap back on, but don't close the top. Now, have a parent light your match and quickly puff it out so it smokes above the bottle. Suck the smoke into the bottle by squeezing the bottle gently and releasing it with the mouth of the bottle in

the smoke. After a few good squeezes, close the cap.

3. Take your shut bottle and squeeze and release a few times.

4. Notice that when you squeeze the bottle, there is no cloud. However, when you release the bottle, a cloud should appear.

TIP: Try mixing up the water temperatures, switching between hot and cold, and see what that does to your cloud.

Discussion

Clouds need only three things to form: water molecules, cloud condensation nuclei (that could mean dust or air pollution), and changes in temperature or air pressure. That's why clouds are more likely to form outside when it's cold.

When you squeeze the bottle, the pressure increases. This causes the temperature inside the bottle to rise. Then, when you release the bottle, the pressure decreases. This causes the temperature inside the bottle to fall and the water molecules to condense and stick together around the smoke. And that's how you make a cloud in a bottle.

EXPERIMENT #10
Make Your Own Motor

There is this old Andraka family saying that there are really only two types of people in the world: those who make the motors and everyone else.

According to legend, that saying has been passed down from generation to generation since Great-Great-Great-Grandpa Arnold Andraka used the motor he invented made from a broken wagon wheel, a quarter tablet of Alka-Seltzer, three rusted coat hangers, and a complicated series of pulleys and levers to sail his mighty vessel across the seven seas.

Okay, maybe that isn't exactly an old Andraka saying. Actually, I just made all that up, but really, this is a *very* cool experiment! And if I actually had a great-great-great-grandpa Arnold Andraka, he would totally agree.

Materials (check your local hardware store)

- Three feet of copper wire
- A magnet
- Two safety pins
- Electrical tape
- A D-cell battery

Procedure

1. Position your D-cell battery on its side. Clip a safety pin to each end. If you have trouble attaching them, use electrical tape so that the head of each safety pin is against the battery's terminals, with the other end of the safety pin (the one with the loop) sticking straight up.

2. Place your magnet on top of your battery.

3. Take your wire and make it into a circle by looping it around a couple of times, leaving the two ends of the wire pointing out in opposite directions. You may want to wrap the ends around the coil a few times to secure it, but be sure there are a few inches sticking out. Make your coil small enough that when you balance the two ends of the coil through the loops on the safety pins, the coil just clears the magnet.

4. Thread the two ends of the wire through each loop in the safety pins. When your coil is in position, give it a push, and the circle of wire should start to rotate.

WARNING: If you use a thin wire, depending on the strength of your current, it can get extremely hot! So be careful.

Discussion

This experiment is a fun way to see how to make a simple version of the motors found in everyday household appliances, tools, and many of the other devices that make your life easier. It's a great experiment for aspiring scientists, because once you get the fundamentals down, you can check online to discover even more complicated motors that you can use to chase around the family pets.

MATH WITH UNCLE TED

LONG-DIVISION TRICK

Here is a handy trick to quickly divide large numbers by 9. Let's try dividing 32,121 by 9.

Start by writing down the first digit of your dividend, in this case 3.

Next, you are going to add 3 to the next number in the dividend, in this case 2. Write down 5.

Now add 5 to the next number in the dividend, 1. Continue adding this way until you reach the end.

$$3\ 2\ 1\ 2\ 1 \div 9$$

$$3\ 5\ 6\ 8 \qquad 9$$

Now, when you are adding the last digit of the dividend, write it off to the side, because this will help you calculate your remainder.

In this case, you are adding 8 and 1, which is 9. 9 goes into 9 once, so you will need to add 1 to your last digit, in this case 8. So your answer is 3,569.

Let's try another. We will divide 153,214 by 9.

$$1\ 5\ 3\ 2\ 1\ 4 \div 9$$

$$\uparrow\uparrow\uparrow\uparrow\uparrow$$

$$1\ 6\ 9\ 11\ 12\qquad 16$$

When you start, enter the first digit of the dividend, which is 1. 1+5 is 6, and then 6+3 is 9. 9+2 is 11, and 11+1 is 12. 12+4 is 16, which you should write to the side because it will help you calculate your remainder.

Since we have some double digits here, let's work from right to left to determine the quotient. Because 9 goes into 16 once, with a remainder of 7, 7 is your remainder and 1 must be added to the ones place of the quotient. 1+12 = 13. Leave the 3 in the ones place of the quotient and add 1 to the previous number, in this case, 11. 11+1 = 12, so the tens digit of the quotient is 2 and the 1 is carried to the hundreds place. 1+9 = 10, so the hundreds place of the quotient is 0 and 1 is added to the thousands place. 6+1 = 7. Your final answer is 17,023 with a remainder of 7.

SQUARING TRICK

Squaring numbers can be tricky. If you're looking for 17^2, for example, you can multiply 10x10 and add it to 7x7, but there is a better way.

First, take the number you wish to square and round it to the nearest multiple of 10. So if you are squaring 27, you would round to 30.

Now, rounding 27 to 30 means adding 3. Subtract the amount that you rounded up by from your original number. In our case, that's 24.

Multiply 24 by 30 and then add 3^2. 3 is the number that you added to 27 to get to the nearest 10.

Because multiplying by 10 is pretty easy (30x24 is just 3x24 with a 0 thrown on the end), this way is a lot faster.

Here our answer is 729: 30x24 is 720 + 3^2 (which is 3x3 = 9) gives you 729.

The rule for this trick is as follows: If you are squaring x, round it to the nearest multiple of 10, and call that x+r. Now take r and subtract it from x, so you have x–r. Multiply these two amounts together (x+r) x (x–r) and then add r^2. The trick works no matter how many digits you have.

This works because $(x+r) \times (x-r) + r^2 = x^2 - rx + rx - r^2 + r^2 = x^2$.

OPEN ACCESS

It turned out that one of the greatest adversities I would have to face during my path to discovery was the simple act of getting my hands on the information that other researchers had already contributed. 90 percent of all scientific articles are wrapped tightly behind paywalls, and buying a subscription that would give you access to a series of articles can cost you thousands of dollars per journal.

I believe that knowledge should not be a commodity and science should not be a luxury. Access to knowledge should be a basic human right.

Without the power of free, online access to scientific and scholarly research articles—a concept called "open access"—we are denied the most natural and efficient way that our society evolves: by building off each other's ideas.

If we are to have any hope of empowering the minds of young scientists to come up with new, creative solutions to the problems of the world, the fight to keep the flow of information free is one of our most important battles.

The time has come to tear down this wall.

Fortunately, at the time of this writing, there is a bipartisan bill called the Fair Access to Science and Technology Research Act (or FASTR) that would require research articles funded by taxpayers to be made freely available online within six months. This bill would help students and established researchers gain access to the articles they need to discover the next breakthrough, accelerate scientific advancement, and improve the lives of people all around the world.

You can tell Congress that you support FASTR and open access by going to the Alliance for Taxpayer Access, www.taxpayeraccess .org, and submitting the form available in their Legislative Action Center at www.congressweb.com/sparc/16.

While all efforts have been made to ensure the accuracy of the information in the following sections as of the date this book was published, it is for informational purposes only. It is not intended to be complete or exhaustive, or a substitute for the advice of a qualified expert or mental health professional.

There are also many fantastic organizations working to help teens who need it. Some of these organizations are included in the following pages. Please note that none of them has endorsed or is otherwise affiliated with me, my story, or this book.

BULLYING AWARENESS

BULLYING FACTS

There are many different kinds of bullying, and none are acceptable. If you see someone being bullied, say something. Research suggests that half of all bullying ends if a bystander intervenes.

Physical—Physical bullying is when a bully hurts someone's body or their possessions. This includes direct attacks, like punching or kicking, and also spitting, tripping, or breaking someone's things.

Verbal—Verbal bullying can be either spoken or written. Name-calling, threatening, insulting, teasing, and offensive remarks all count. Verbal bullying can also include inappropriate sexual comments.

Social—This type of bullying is usually more indirect. Social bullying includes spreading rumors about someone, exclusion, embarrassing someone in public, or even sending abusive mail.

Cyberbullying—This is bullying that happens online or electronically. Cyberbullying includes sending hurtful text messages, emails, phone calls, instant messages, unwanted pictures, videos, or website links.[1] [2]

BULLYING TIPS

What do you do if you're being bullied? Well, this is what I'd tell middle school Jack:

Talk to your parents.

Looking back, I should have gone to my parents earlier. I think that would have saved me so much pain. If haters are making you so miserable that you find yourself wishing entire years of your life away, that might mean it's time to swallow your pride and call in the reinforcements.

If you are waiting for the perfect time to have this conversation, forget it. Know that nothing about the conversation will be easy. Just try to find someplace where there aren't any distractions and you have their complete attention. Remember, your parents want to see you grow up and be happy, not being tortured. And most important, if it gets really bad, parents are the only ones who have the power to remove you from that negative environment and place you in a

---

1. stopbullying.gov, www.stopbullying.gov/what-is-bullying/definition

2. National Centre Against Bullying, www.ncab.org.au/parents/typesofbullying

more positive one where you can have the opportunity to pursue the things that make you happy.

Give social media a break.

I know a lot of parents advise their kids to just stay offline, but that isn't always realistic today. For a young person, cutting off connections to social media can mean severing ties with their entire social circle. If you aren't willing to delete your Facebook profile, at least change your privacy settings so you can control who has permission to see your profile. If that doesn't work, you may have to put your profile in hibernation mode and reactivate your account later.

Twitter is a different story. If a cyber-hater is riding you on Twitter, it can be impossible to block mentions or interactions. In those cases, your only option might be to completely delete your account, at least until Twitter take steps to upgrade its privacy settings.

If nothing else works, change schools.

Today, more than ever, there are more and more quality learning opportunities, whether it be through the expansion of charters or great new online schools. By changing schools you aren't running away from your problems. You are choosing to take yourself out of a negative environment and place yourself in a positive one.

I understand that this probably isn't the answer most of you wanted or expected, but if you are serious about getting through those rough years so you can achieve something special with your life, sometimes you are going to have to take a more unconventional route.

If you find yourself running out of options and need a place to turn, remember that there is always hope.

LGBTQ AWARENESS

LGBTQ stands for lesbian, gay, bisexual, transgender, and queer. LGBTQ teens like me are often teased or harassed for being different.

LGBTQ BULLYING FACTS

- Nine out of ten people who identify as LGBTQ have reported bullying at school because of their sexual orientation.

- Half of those people have been victims of physical bullying, and a quarter have been physically assaulted.

- 64 percent of LGBTQ students feel unsafe at school because of their sexual orientation. 44 percent feel unsafe at school because of gender identification.

- 32 percent of LGBTQ students have not gone to school for at least a day because they felt unsafe.[3]

---

3. www.nobullying.com/lgbt-bullying-statistics

LGBTQ RESOURCES

The It Gets Better Project

This project helps illustrate that life really does get better for LGBTQ youth. View a collection of videos and resources from LGBTQ adults and allies around the world at www.itgetsbetter.org.

GLBT National Help Center

No matter your age, you can get advice, support, and resources from peers throughout the United States at www.glbtnationalhelpcenter.org.

The Trevor Project

This is the leading national organization for crisis intervention and suicide prevention for LGBTQ youth between the ages of thirteen and twenty-four. You can visit their website at www.thetrevorproject .org or call them at 866-488-7386.

SUICIDE PREVENTION

Suicide is the third leading cause of death for fifteen- to twenty-four-year-olds. That means more teens die every year from suicide than from terminal illness—way more than pancreatic cancer. On average, teens who commit suicide have twenty-five failed attempts before doing so. That's twenty-five times (at least) to get help.

If you are having thoughts about suicide, there are people you can talk to.

Talk to someone. Talk to your parents, your teachers, a trusted adult. They're here to help you and they're here to make sure you're here for a long time, too.

You can also always call the National Suicide Prevention Lifeline at 1-800-273-8255. They take calls 24/7.

Just remember, you are not alone.